Hashimoto's Thyroiditis:
Lifestyle Interventions for Finding and Treating the Root Cause

Izabella Wentz, PharmD, FASCP

with Marta Nowosadzka, MD

Disclaimer

The medical information in this book is provided as an educational resource only, and is not intended to be used or relied upon for any diagnostic or treatment purposes. This information should not be used as a substitute for professional diagnosis and treatment.

The lifestyle interventions discussed in this book should not be used as a substitute for conventional medical therapy.

Furthermore, none of the statements in this book have been evaluated by the Food and Drug Administration.

Please consult your health-care provider before making any health-care decisions or for guidance about a specific medical condition.

DEDICATION

This book is dedicated to all of the women and men who have Hashimoto's Thyroiditis and other autoimmune conditions. I hope that this book will empower you with the necessary knowledge to recover your health. Be well!

CONTENTS

ACKNOWLEDGMENTS

First and foremost, I would like to thank my loving husband Michael, who has supported me through this whole process. Thank you, honey, for sticking with me when I was bloated, grumpy, and lethargic. Thank you for the extra warmth when I was inconsolably cold. And thank you for trying all of my new diets with me. Most of all, thank you for loving me, and for listening to my ever-evolving theories on my thyroid health. I am so lucky to have you and love you infinitely!

My brilliant mom, the best doctor I have ever had, for always believing in me and giving me so many wonderful ideas. We have spent countless hours bouncing health-care theories off one another with much benefit. Thank you for the reminders to keep moving forward.

My dad and my brother, for your support and effort to make me feel better.

To my wonderful friends April and Wendy, for your encouragement, support, and willingness to listen to all of my nontraditional theories.

I am grateful to be living in the digital age, when one can find hope and reassurance in stories of those undergoing similar circumstances. Thank you for sharing your stories!

Last but not least, I want to thank all of the wonderful clinicians I have had the pleasure of meeting. Each has given me one or more pieces to this puzzle, and provided me with directions to the next destination in my journey. I especially want to thank Elena Koles, MD, PhD, my personal physician, for guiding me along my journey and encouraging me to be an active member of my healthcare team.

"You must be the change you want to see in the world." — Gandhi

1: INTRODUCTION

Why Focus On Hashimoto's?

The easiest answer to this question is that I was diagnosed with Hashimoto's thyroiditis during a routine physical at age 27.

As a pharmacist, I was trained about the pathophysiology of diseases, as well therapeutic treatments. My professors always stressed lifestyle interventions to reduce the need for medications and to prevent disease progression.

People with hypertension were told to eat a low-sodium diet, people with high cholesterol were supposed to reduce their fat intake, and Type 2 diabetics could essentially reverse their condition by eating foods with low glycemic indexes and by losing weight.

In mild cases of most chronic conditions, I was always taught to recommend lifestyle interventions first, followed by medication therapy if the interventions were unsuccessful, or if the patient was not willing to change.

In advanced cases, and if the benefits of medications outweighed the risks, the patients would be started on medications **in conjunction** with lifestyle interventions.

We also learned that patients should be monitored as they made progress toward their goals to see if medication therapy was still warranted.

Thus, I was perplexed that there were no mainstream lifestyle interventions for Hashimoto's, or any autoimmune conditions, for that matter. The only intervention for Hashimoto's that was recommended by my endocrinologist was pharmacological one, to start taking a supplemental thyroid hormone such as Synthroid®, one of the most commonly prescribed medications in the United States.

While I was prepared to start taking Synthroid® after having a gradual decrease of thyroid hormone production as I aged well into my 90s, I didn't feel this medication was sufficient as the sole treatment for an autoimmune condition. The supplemental hormone did not stop the destruction of the thyroid gland by the immune system. It simply added more hormone when the thyroid was too damaged to produce it on its own. It was like pouring water into a leaky bucket without plugging up the holes that were causing the leak.

Furthermore, I was only 27! I just got married, started my dream job, moved to a house by the beach in Los Angeles ... this was not right.

I am a firm believer in cause and effect, and it did not make sense to me that this disorder just happened out of nowhere. On top of it all, I had been suffering from severe digestive troubles for many years, was chronically fatigued, and was experiencing profuse hair loss. It seemed unnatural to me to do nothing as a part of my body was being destroyed. It didn't make sense. Those who know me will attest that I can be quite stubborn when I feel that I have been wronged.

One can think that the world is unfair and ponder the many reasons for the lack of lifestyle interventions, but focusing on the problem never seems to yield a solution.

But perhaps, I thought to myself, if I could make connections among all of my symptoms, then maybe I could find and treat the root cause of my condition, and hopefully my story will inspire others to do the same.

Sometimes we have to be the change we want to happen, and hope that the medical establishment will take note and promote further research.

While this book is based on research, and results have been reproduced, many of the statements in this book are based my own personal observations and experience. Furthermore, everyone is unique and the interventions that worked for me may not work for others.

Above all I strive first to do no harm, so please be sure to listen to your own body and seek medical care when necessary. Be sure that if you are taking thyroid hormone your levels are monitored on a regular basis (i.e., every six to twelve weeks), as your condition may change after implementing lifestyle interventions.

The bottom line: While this book may not help everyone find and treat the root cause of their condition, it will describe how people with Hashimoto's hypothyroidism can feel better, lead a healthier lifestyle, and will hopefully inspire you the reader to take charge of your own health.

October 6, 2009

Me: a 27-year-old woman, passionate about my career, newly wed, proud owner of an adorable Pomeranian, frugal (yet trendy and stylish), amateur chef, aspiring cosmetic chemist, family oriented, ex-smoker, non-drinker, yoga enthusiast, scrapbook lover, health-care professional ... with Hashimoto's thyroiditis.

What does Hashimoto's mean to you? To me, it meant losing my hair, feeling exhausted, anxious, cold, and forgetful (a.k.a. the infamous "brain fog"), followed by pain and numbness in both of my arms.

To some, Hashimoto's may mean recurrent miscarriages, an inability to lose weight despite diet and exercise, depression, constipation, and years of frustration.

To others, it may mean pale skin, premature aging, feeling lethargic, unmotivated, sluggish …

I suspect that my journey with Hashimoto's, like for many of you, began many years before diagnosis, which in my case was in 2009.

Without going into too much detail, the first of the crucial defining moments in my disease development may have started during my undergraduate studies at the University of Illinois. Due to the communal living setting of dormitories (and less than stellar hygiene habits of most college students) I had recurrent strep throat infections and even contracted mononucleosis, a viral infection caused by the Epstein-Barr Virus (EBV), which is implicated in triggering many autoimmune conditions. I received multiple courses of antibiotics as well as flu shots (which may be associated with EBV infections), and started birth control for menstrual cramps.

It is my belief that this combination had a profound impact on my gut flora, and thus my immune system—the significance of which you will learn in the next few chapters.

Up until the middle half of my freshman year in college, I used to be an early riser who only needed six to eight hours of sleep. I woke up energetic and ready to face the day each morning.

However, after one particularly nasty sore throat, I just could not get enough sleep, no matter what time I went to bed! I once arrived thirty minutes late to an 8 a.m. exam, having just woken after sleeping for sixteen hours straight (I had lain down for a quick nap the day before at 4 p.m.).

A previously straight-A student, I barely passed my classes that semester. Discouraged, I spent the summer after my freshman year going to bed at 9 p.m. only to wake up exhausted around 1 or 2 p.m. the next day.

Within a few months, my need for sleep began to subside, however, I felt that I never fully recovered since that time, requiring much more sleep than I had prior to the mono infection.

Two years later, during the first year of my pharmacy studies, I required a series of immunizations in order to be allowed to start my clinical rotations, and developed irritable bowel syndrome (IBS) with diarrhea, which seemed to be triggered by soy lecithin. Upon cutting out soy lecithin-containing foods, my symptoms reduced from daily to once or twice per week. Further elimination of red meat eliminated the symptoms.

A bout of urinary tract, yeast, and throat infections, as well as acne the following year, led to the use of additional antibiotics.

My lifestyle was filled with fast food, late-night study sessions, caffeine, stress, and virtually no time for myself.

Towards the end of my fourth year of pharmacy school, I started noticing an onset of anxiety symptoms. I attributed the anxiety to the changes I was undergoing at the time: graduating, taking board exams, getting engaged, moving to a new city, finding a new job…

The following year, I came down with a terrible viral infection with the hacking, lungs-coming-out kind of cough. The lack of energy went away after a few days of missed work and lying around at home, but the cough lingered. I would wake up in the middle of the night choking. I often would have uncontrollable fits of coughing while counseling patients at the pharmacy where I worked. One day I was coughing so hard I vomited in a trash can in the bathroom.

"Are you pregnant?" one of the clerks asked with an assuming smile.

"No, I take pills for that," I replied.

Being a pharmacist, I tried every over-the-counter cough syrup that was available at the drug store where I worked. The cough persisted. I tried Claritin®, Zyrtec®, Allegra®, Flonase®, Albuterol .... none of those helped, either! I ended up seeing an allergy specialist after a primary care doctor ran a blood allergy test that showed that— yikes!—I was allergic to dogs!

The allergy specialist ran more detailed tests. First was the "itchy skin" test, also known as the scratch test, where a nurse scratches your back with a pin that contains small amounts of allergen and watches for a reaction. It turned out that I was allergic to—wait for it—everything! Horses (which might explain my irrational fear of them), dogs (although I've had dogs most of my life, while the cough had just started), trees (all of the ones native to California), and grass (strangely, I was more allergic to grass than I was to histamine).

I was started on Singulair®, Xyzal®, and Nasonex®, but they did not help the cough. The second test was called a barium swallow, where you swallow a whole bunch of chalky liquid so the doctor can image your esophagus. (Side effect: white poop!)

I received a diagnosis of a small sliding hiatal hernia with spontaneous reflux, and thus gastro esophageal reflux disease (GERD), commonly known as acid reflux.

I was actually relieved to have a diagnosis! Finally, an answer, although I was somewhat puzzled as I didn't have any of the typical symptoms of GERD that we learned about in school.

I started on Aciphex®, an acid-suppressing medication used for GERD, and followed up with a gastrointestinal specialist. He said "Take two a day for a few months and call me for refills".

Soon after taking the Aciphex®, I actually developed symptoms of GERD. The cough continued. I decided to discontinue the Aciphex®, and implemented anti-reflux dietary changes and began to sleep pretty much upright. I also started taking Pepcid®, another medication for reflux, Mylanta®, and drinking ginger tea. I believe that these medications further contributed to a change in gut flora.

Later that summer, I traveled to Poland with my family and experienced almost daily food poisoning with severe diarrhea for two weeks—another strike against my gut flora. After my return to the U.S., I began to notice hair loss, but I dismissed it on the belief that it must have been all in my head (no pun intended). A few months later, it was that time of year again to get a full physical.

<u>September 2009</u>
Thyroid antibodies = 2000
TSH = 7.88
Normal T3 and T4

Diagnosis: Hashimoto's Thyroiditis and Subclinical Hypothyroidism

I was also told I had a possible mitral valve prolapse or murmur that needed to be checked out by a cardiologist.

I was in shock and disbelief.

I read up about the symptoms of hypothyroidism, or an underactive thyroid, and perhaps I had some of them, but the symptoms were so nonspecific that I rationalized all of them away to stress, work, getting older and everyday life worries.

While it was true that I slept for more than twelve hours each night, I had just grown to live with it, and decided that it was the new normal for me. Additionally, I had been checked for anemia, thyroid disorders, and other common reasons for fatigue a few years back when living in Arizona, and was told everything was fine.

Quite frankly, I was shocked that I had hypothyroidism and not hyperthyroidism. In the textbooks I had from pharmacy school, people who had underactive thyroids were overweight and sluggish. This clinical picture did not fit me.

I've always had cold intolerance, but I attributed that to my low body fat. Weight gain? Not me.

Depression? Not at all, this was the happiest I had been in my life.

Slow, sluggish? Not me! Have you seen me running around at work??

While I did sleep for more than twelve hours every night, I was very anxious, thin, and tired but wired. If anything, I thought, an overactive thyroid (hyperthyroidism) seemed to fit me better.

What I came to later understand is that as the thyroid antibodies produced in autoimmune thyroiditis were attacking my thyroid, packets of hormone were released into my blood stream, causing symptoms of an overactive thyroid in addition to those of the underactive thyroid. The best of both worlds.

Once the shock settled, I found out that lifelong thyroid medications are recommended, and that untreated Hashimoto's can lead to serious manifestations such as heart disease, severe weight gain, and infertility. As a newlywed, the last one was especially hard to swallow.

Endocrinologists were divided on whether to start thyroid hormones or wait in case of subclinical hypothyroidism. Additionally, most medical websites stated that nothing could be done for the autoimmune destruction of the gland.

But I knew in my heart of hearts (or perhaps it was my gut), that waiting around while a part of my body destroyed itself just couldn't be right. I decided to use the scientific literature review skills gained during courses in pharmacy school to look for any new research or studies about Hashimoto's.

Within a couple of hours, I was able to find the following encouraging information:

- Selenium 200-300 mcg daily has been shown to reduce anti-thyroid antibodies by 20%-50%, over one year. And yes it was a statistically significant study, for you statistics buffs! (p value <0.000005)[1]
- Thyroid supplementation may be used with subclinical hypothyroidism to improve outcomes.[2]
- Strict adherence to a gluten-free diet normalized subclinical hypothyroidism in those with celiac disease [3]

I also decided to search information on medical boards where patients would share their experiences. In my work as a clinical consulting pharmacist, I often examined these types of sites to gain insight about patient perspectives on the effectiveness of various medications. Many times, these sites contained information that had not yet been described in the scientific and mainstream literature and was still experimental.

I was excited to read a testimonial that stated: "Acupuncture eliminated my need for levothyroid (I was up to 300 mcg per day); and I no longer test positive for anti-thyroid antibodies."[4]

Unfortunately, my insurance did not cover acupuncture, but what did

I have to lose (other than money, of course)? I decided to give it a shot. I also scheduled appointments with an endocrine specialist, cardiologist, and gynecologist. I felt 27 going on 72.

Over the next three years, I spent an enormous amount of time and money to heal myself. I have read various books, spent countless hours researching medical journals, health blogs, and making myself a human guinea pig.

I have researched, considered, and/or tried various interventions to heal my Hashimoto's, including:

- Acupuncture
- Low-dose Naltrexone
- Fluoride-free toothpaste
- Kombucha tea
- Adaptogens
- Expensive thyroid specialists
- Compounded thyroid medications
- Synthroid® (levothyroxine)
- Armour® thyroid
- Goiterogen avoidance
- Seaweed snacks
- Alkalizing the body
- Medicinal herbs
- Dr. Hyman's protocol
- Dr. Brownstein's protocol
- Dr. Kharazzian's protocol
- Dr. Haskell's protocol
- Psychic consultation
- Endocrinologist
- Chiropractor
- Selenium supplementation
- Gluten-free/dairy-free/soy-free diet
- Caveman/Paleo diet

- GAPS/SCD diet
- Body Ecology Diet
- Probiotics
- Iodine consumption/avoidance
- Coconut virgin oil
- A pharmacy's worth of various vitamins and supplements
- Detoxification
- Glandulars
- Protomorphogens
- Marshall Protocol
- Immune balancing
- Juicing
- Fermented foods
- Treating infections

I became obsessed with finding the answer, and as those who know me can confirm, I am very stubborn and determined to get my way.

PROTEIN: MY AHA! MOMENT

Protein indigestion/malabsorption

When I first became chronically exhausted, I would sleep as long as possible. This was much easier as a college student. Unfortunately, it led to having a less than stellar GPA. But I soon learned to compensate. I would sleep all day, and then stay up to study all night to take my exams at 7:30 a.m., come home, and sleep more.

Other times, when I had to wake up with less than ten hours of sleep, I would often be struck with diarrhea. With the help of a supervising pharmacist, I was able to connect the diarrhea to protein shakes that contained soy lecithin. Red meat was also a culprit in causing gastrointestinal distress, as was lack of adequate sleep.

I remember saying to my mom, "It's like I need to sleep so that my body can process everything I ate, when I wake up too early it's still not processed." She suspected lactose intolerance. "It can't be," I thought. "Why would it just start all of a sudden?"

Fast forward to the future. I started taking Betaine with Pepsin on Friday, February 10, 2012, one capsule with each meal containing protein. I was surprised to wake up the following morning at 8 am without an alarm. I had been dragging myself out of bed after 10 most mornings when I did not have to work. Strangely, I continued to feel energetic all day. I even stayed awake when my usually much more energetic husband took a nap. With a friend's wedding fast approaching and having barely exercised in the last year, I had also started doing P90X on that same Friday.

I wondered if my new energy was due to the exercise or to the enzymes. Happily, I continued both, and thought I should test my theory at some point. Meanwhile, things became easier, and all of a sudden, I felt that I had a surplus of time. I felt more at ease going to bed and even had time to meditate, something that I had been wanting to do for years!

As the week went on, I felt myself having more and more energy, and actually became more outgoing and talkative. Additionally, the mental fog was completely lifted, and I could come up with all sorts of clever words quickly. My co-workers commented on my good mood at work. My husband noticed that my sense of humor even improved. I felt like myself again, the self that I had not seen for almost ten years.

I woke up one day at 5:17 a.m. and decided to start writing this book. I had always loved writing, and even took a workshop about writing a novel in 2007. The instructor suggested that working people have the best chance of writing a book by waking up two hours prior to their usual rising time to write. With a full-time job and responsibilities, I thought becoming an author would be impossible, and I gave up that dream. But now, here I was ... doing the impossible. Certainly, if I could wake up energized after only six hours of sleep after feeling chronically exhausted for ten years I could easily overcome Hashimoto's and then write a book about it!

But the journey did not stop there. The energetic feeling only lasted a few weeks, and unfortunately, I have had many setbacks before I found something that worked for me. But I never forgot how great it was to finally feel normal and kept pushing on and fighting. After much perseverance, time, and trial and error, I can finally say that I was successful and my Hashimoto's is in remission.

I am going to share my research and rationale for the root cause and treatment of Hashimoto's based on what finally worked for me, with the hope that it may also work for some of my readers. I am also going to share the process of how I came to find my root cause, so that hopefully, my readers will be inspired to find theirs using a similar methodology.

The next three chapters will summarize the conventional knowledge about Hashimoto's that most physicians learn during their training in medical school. This knowledge is about fifteen to twenty years behind the knowledge that will be presented in subsequent chapters, but will serve as a great starting point for expanding your knowledge about Hashimoto's Thyroiditis.

PART I: UNDERSTANDING HASHIMOTO'S

"Knowledge will bring you the opportunity to make a difference." – Claire Fagin

2. BASIC THYROID KNOWLEDGE

So What the Heck is a Thyroid?

The thyroid gland is a butterfly-shaped organ that is located in the neck below the Adam's apple.

The thyroid produces thyroid hormones that affect the function of just about every organ system in the human body.

Thyroid hormones are responsible for the very important role of stimulating the metabolism of the foods we eat, and extracting vitamins and producing energy from food. They are also vital to the production of other hormones as well as the growth and development of our nervous system.

The thyroid has been called the "thermostat" of our body, as it maintains our temperature. Indirectly, thyroid function affects every reaction in the human body, as the temperature has to be just right for these reactions to take place properly. [15]

Thyroid Hormone Production

The thyroid gland has multiple small narrow cavities called follicles that are filled with a clear material known as thyroglobulin (sometimes called colloid) that is produced by a layer of thyroid epithelial cells known as thyrocytes. This material contains tyrosine, an amino acid that is a starting material used for thyroid hormone synthesis. Thyroglobulin functions as a reservoir for materials used in thyroid production, including the storage of iodine.

Iodide absorbed from food circulates in our blood and is absorbed into the thyroid gland where it must be converted into a form usable by the body through an oxidation process. The enzyme Thyroid PerOxidase (TPO) converts iodide to the active iodine making hydrogen peroxide as a byproduct. The reactive iodine is now ready to attach to other molecules, and attaches to the amino acid tyrosine in thyroglobulin through a process known as "iodination."

During iodination, each molecule of tyrosine combines with one or two iodine molecules, resulting in either monoiodotyrosine (T1) or diiodotyrosine (T2). The molecules then bond to form either triiodothyronine (T3, thyroglobulin with three iodine molecules) or thyroxine (T4, thyroglobulin with four iodine molecules).

T1+T2=T3 or T2+T2=T4

Of the four iodinated molecules, only T3 and T4 are considered to be biologically active in the body. However, Thyroxine (T4) is known as pro-hormone, and is 300% less biologically active than T3. Thus, Triiodothyronine (T3) is the main biologically active thyroid hormone. These molecules are stored in thyroid follicles until they are needed.

Twenty percent of T3 comes from thyroid secretion, while the remaining 80% comes from T4 when T4 is converted to T3 through the deiodination process (which removes one iodine molecule) in peripheral organs like the liver and kidney. Zinc is required to convert T4 to T3.

Low levels of T3 and T4 signal release of TSH (Thyroid Stimulating Hormone), while high levels of circulating T3 and T4 stop the release of TSH. In people with normal thyroid function, TSH levels may fluctuate in times when more thyroid hormone is consumed, such as in stress, illness, lack of sleep, pregnancy, or low temperatures. [15]

Thyroid Hormone Disorders

Thyroid hormone disorders can be classified as those resulting in inadequate thyroid hormone production, or hypothyroidism, as well as an overabundance of thyroid hormone production, or hyperthyroidism.

Hypothyroidism

Some of the more common symptoms of hypothyroidism, or deficiency of thyroid hormone, include slower metabolism leading to gaining weight, forgetfulness, feeling cold or cold intolerance, depression, fatigue, dry skin, constipation, loss of ambition, hair loss, muscle cramps, stiffness, joint pain, a loss of the outer third eyebrow, menstrual irregularities, infertility and weakness.

Iodine deficiency versus Hashimoto's

When there is a deficiency in the building blocks required to make thyroid hormone (iodide, selenium, zinc, tyrosine), TSH is triggered to signal additional production of TPO to start converting the stored iodide to a usable form, (this also results in hydrogen peroxide production). If no iodide is available, an enlargement of the thyroid gland will result in the body's attempt to try to increase thyroid hormone production by compensating through increasing the size of thyroid cells. The enlargement is known as a goiter.

Iodine deficiency can cause hypothyroidism and goiter and is the leading cause of hypothyroidism in many underdeveloped countries. However, in the United States and many European countries that add iodine to salt or other foods, Hashimoto's is the leading cause of hypothyroidism, and not iodine deficiency. In fact, Hashimoto's is responsible for 90% of cases of hypothyroidism in the U.S.A

Additional causes of hypothyroidism include silent (or painless) thyroiditis and postpartum thyroiditis, both of which are associated with antibody production but resolve on their own with a resolution of antibodies and return to normal thyroid function. In some cases, these conditions may be followed years later by Hashimoto's. Silent thyroiditis has been associated with seasonal allergies, viral infections and vigorous neck massage. The trigger for postpartum thyroiditis is pregnancy. Perhaps these two conditions are examples of the beginning of an autoimmune response that becomes extinguished once the triggers are removed. [1,2,3,13]

<u>Do you have an enlarged thyroid?</u> [5]

Check your Neck!

You can examine your own thyroid with a handheld mirror and glass of water. The thyroid gland is located at the base on the neck, below your Adam's apple.

1. Hold the mirror in your hand and look at the area of the neck below you Adam's apple and immediately above your collarbone. (Don't confuse the Adam's apple with the thyroid, the thyroid is further down).
2. While still looking in the mirror, tip your head back, and take a drink of water from your glass.
3. As you swallow, look at your neck. Be aware of bulges or protrusions as you swallow.
4. If you see any bulges or protrusion, you may have an enlarged thyroid gland or thyroid nodule. [5]

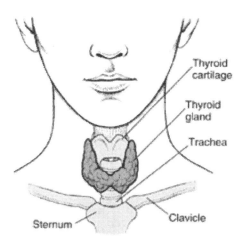

Figure 1: Illustration of the Thyroid Gland

From The Merck Manual of Medical Information - Second Home Edition, p. 948, edited by Mark H. Beers. Copyright © 2003 by Merck & Co., Inc., Whitehouse Station, NJ. Available at: http://www.merck.com/mmhe/sec13/ch163/ch163a.html Accessed March 29, 2013

Hyperthyroidism

Hyperthyroidism, or an overabundance of thyroid hormone has a stimulatory effect. Classical symptoms include weight loss, palpitations, anxiety, eye bulging, tremors, irritability, menstrual disturbances, fatigue, heat intolerance, and increased appetite. Patients may often have hair loss.

Hyperthyroidism is usually caused by a related autoimmune condition called Graves' disease where antibodies to the TSH Receptor are present. Graves' can sometimes evolve into Hashimoto's and vice versa, and the two disorders seem to be closely related.

Hashimoto's Thyroiditis

Hashimoto's Thyroiditis is an autoimmune condition that results in destruction of the thyroid gland. This damage eventually leads to inadequate thyroid hormone production, or hypothyroidism. Hashimoto's is the most common cause of hypothyroidism in the United States, and accounts for 90% of cases of hypothyroidism.

Hashimoto's thyroiditis is also known as chronic thyroiditis, lymphocytic thyroiditis, lymphadenoid goiter, and recently autoimmune thyroiditis. This condition was first described in 1912 by a Japanese physician, Hakuro Hashimoto, who first called it struma lymphomatosa.

Hashimoto's usually begins as a gradual enlargement of the thyroid gland, which can sometimes be noticeable to the patient on self-examination. It can be accompanied by hoarseness or breathing difficulty and occasionally patients may experience tenderness or pain.

When the damage to the gland is just beginning, the body compensates and produces more hormone, and thus the hormone levels are kept within "normal" ranges, however the person may start noticing symptoms of hypothyroidism. Mild hypothyroidism may be noticed in some patients, while in others, thyrotoxicosis (too much thyroid hormone) can be present. This beginning stage is a described as a "subclinical" hypothyroidism. Subclinical hypothyroidism is defined as an increased TSH, but "normal" T4 and T3.

Progressively, as more thyroid tissue is destroyed, the thyroid loses its ability to compensate and the person becomes deficient in thyroid hormone. Eventually, this results in a complete loss of ability to produce thyroid hormone by the gland (atrophic thyroiditis), which is considered as the end stage of Hashimoto's thyroiditis.

In Hashimoto's two types of self reactive antibodies can be seen. More than 90% of people with Hashimoto's have thyroid peroxidase antibodies (TPOAb), and about 80% of people with Hashimoto's have thyroglobulin antibodies (TgAb). [1, 14]

Prevalence

Hashimoto's affects up to 10% of the population in the U.S., and prevalence increases with age. Hashimoto's affects predominantly women at a rate of seven women for every one man with Hashimoto's. Hormonal fluctuation may contribute to the development of Hashimoto's and peak effects are seen around puberty, pregnancy and menopause. Up to 20% of women may have TPO antibodies indicative of Hashimoto's. There seems to be a higher incidence of this condition in Caucasians and Japanese compared to individuals of African or Mexican descent. [1, 14]

Thyroid Changes in Hashimoto's

If we were to look at the thyroid gland in Hashimoto's under a microscope, we can observe thyroid cell destruction, a pooling of white blood cells and scarring of thyroid tissue. The thyroid cells are slightly larger. In contrast, thyroglobulin, the usually present reservoir of thyroid hormones and raw materials for hormone production is significantly shrunken.

Ultrasound of the thyroid usually shows an enlarged gland with normal texture and a characteristic picture with a low reflection of the ultrasound waves (low echogenicity), which means that the tissue has become less solid and more rubbery. These changes are seen on the entire lobe or gland. [14]

Symptoms of Hashimoto's

People with Hashimoto's may experience BOTH hypothyroid and hyperthyroid symptoms because as the thyroid cells are destroyed, stored hormones are released into the circulation causing a toxic level of thyroid hormone in the body, also known as thyrotoxicosis or Hashitoxicosis.

Eventually, the stored thyroid may become depleted and due to thyroid cell damage, the person is no longer able to produce enough hormones. At this time, hypothyroidism develops.

Complications

One fourth of patients may experience physical symptoms such as chest pain and/or joint pain. Hypothyroidism also puts people at an increased risk of heart disease.

Hashimoto's patients are three times more likely to develop thyroid cancer compared to people without the condition.

Pregnancy

Sadly, women with positive TPO antibodies have an increased risk of miscarriage, and women who have an underactive thyroid during pregnancy are at risk of delivering an intellectually disabled child.[16,17,18]

Thyroid screening is not a routine test performed until later in life, so many women don't discover that they have Hashimoto's until they have experienced recurrent miscarriages.

Remission of Hashimoto's with loss of goiter, hypothyroidism, and serum antibodies has been reported in pregnancy, with a relapse after delivery. Usually the antibodies decrease during pregnancy. Pregnancy has also been identified as a trigger for Hashimoto's, and also causes a condition known as postpartum thyroiditis, which is self-limiting in 80% of cases, but develops into Hashimoto's in 20% of cases.

Risk factors

There is a genetic predisposition to developing Hashimoto's, and it tends to run in families. Thus, relatives of those with Hashimoto's are at risk. Hashimoto's thyroiditis can occur in two varieties: an organ wasting form (atrophic) associated with HLA-DR3 gene inheritance and enlarged thyroid (goiterous form) through HLA-DR5 inheritance. These genes are very common in the Caucasian population.

Well established environmental triggers for developing Hashimoto's in those who are genetically predisposed include iodine intake, bacterial and viral infections, hormonal imbalances, toxins, as well as therapy with certain types of medications. Cigarette smoking, surprisingly, has been associated with a reduced risk of Hashimoto's.

It's interesting to note that in people with Hashimoto's, only 50% of their identical twins presented with thyroid antibodies, meaning that genes alone are not the be all end all and that environmental triggers are extremely important. [1]

Co-occurring Conditions

Hashimoto's may be associated with other autoimmune diseases like Type 1 diabetes mellitus, multiple sclerosis, rheumatoid arthritis, celiac disease, lupus, Addison's disease, pernicious anemia and hypoparathyroidism. Polyglandular autoimmunity is a medical term used to describe when one person has two or more autoimmune diseases. [1]

DIAGNOSIS

Tests for Hashimoto's

Thyroid ultrasounds as well as blood tests are used to diagnose Hashimoto's. Laboratory tests are available to check thyroid function, and autoimmune thyroid markers. If we were to perform blood tests in advanced untreated Hashimoto's, we would find an elevated TSH, and low levels of T3 and T4. Thyroid antibodies are also found in most cases of Hashimoto's.

Screening Test

TSH is used as a screening test for thyroid function, however it may not always catch thyroid abnormalities. TSH does not become permanently elevated until the Hashimoto's is advanced. Thus, people may have a normal TSH for many years while experiencing the unpleasant thyroid symptoms. They will present to their physicians with complaints of weight gain, fatigue, and other thyroid symptoms and will be told that their thyroid tests were normal. However, TSH levels can fluctuate throughout the day, and the body often compensates by shifting energy away from metabolism and other body functions as long as it can, and this test will miss many cases of hypothyroidism.

Untreated hypothyroidism eventually results in an abnormally elevated TSH. In contrast untreated hyperthyroidism results in an abnormally low TSH. A person with Hashimoto's may fluctuate between the two extremes but still have "normal" readings.

This is because when the level of thyroid hormones is low, TSH is released to order the body to compensate and make more hormone.

When TSH is released, it signals the body to produce more hydrogen peroxide. Thyroid hormone production requires iodide from food to be oxidized into iodine, a molecule that can attach to tyrosine and make thyroid hormone. Hydrogen peroxide is required for this conversion, and is a reactive oxygen species and can cause tissue damage when not enough antioxidants are present. Glutathione peroxidase is the antioxidant that is responsible for neutralizing hydrogen peroxide. Selenium is a component of this antioxidant, and is required for proper thyroid function.

$$Iodide(from\ food) + Hydrogen\ Peroxide \rightarrow Iodine$$

Most conventional physicians use the TSH screening test to determine if one has a thyroid disorder, however, this can often times be misleading, as levels of circulating hormones may fluctuate at different times, such as in Hashimoto's, the person affected may fluctuate between highs and lows.

Additionally, when scientists first set the "normal" ranges of TSH for healthy individuals, they inadvertently included elderly patients and others with compromised thyroid function in the calculations leading to an overly lax reference range. As a result, people with underactive thyroid hormones were often told that their thyroid tests were "normal," based on this skewed reference range.

In recent years, The National Academy of Clinical Biochemists indicated that 95% of individuals without thyroid disease have TSH concentrations below 2.5 µIU/L, and a new normal reference range was defined by the American College of Clinical Endocrinologists to be between 0.3- 3.0 µIU/ml.[2]

However, most labs have not adjusted that range in the reports they provide to physicians, and have kept ranges as lax as 0.2-8.0 µIU/ml. Most physicians only look for values outside of the "normal" reference range provided by the labs, and may not be familiar with the new guidelines. Many physicians may miss the patients who are showing an elevated TSH. This is one reason why patients should always ask their physicians for a copy of any lab results.

Functional medicine practitioners have further defined that normal reference ranges should be between 1 and 2 μIU/ml, for a healthy person not taking thyroid medications.

It's important to remember that reference ranges may not be applicable to everyone. What is normal for one person may be abnormal for the next. Reference ranges take into account the average values of 95% of the population. Thus, not everyone falls within the "normal" reference range. If you are in the other 5%, you may experience symptoms of hypothyroidism or hyperthyroidism with TSH values that are considered normal. All clinicians are taught the old adage "treat the patient and not the lab tests," but unfortunately not many conventional doctors seem to follow this advice.

Even with all of the redefined normal ranges, TSH screening only catches the late stage of Hashimoto's as in the beginning stages of thyroid dysfunction, the body is still able to compensate.

Hormone tests

T4 (Thyroxine) and T3 (Triiodothyronine) are the two main thyroid hormones. T4 is known as pro-hormone, and is 300% less biologically active than T3. T3 is the main biologically active thyroid hormone.

There are two ways to test the thyroid hormones. Total hormone levels measure all of the thyroid hormones in the body, but they may not paint an accurate picture of the situation. "Free" hormone levels measure the hormone that is available to do its job in the body. Thus, tests for Free T4 and Free T3 are recommended.

Some clinicians may only test for T4, but T3 is also important to test, as some individuals may not be converting the T4 to the active T3 properly. Some individuals may have a normal T4, but a low T3 level.

Reverse T3 (rT3) is also a test that can be done to see how much of the free active T3 is able to bind at thyroid receptors. RT3 is produced in stressful situations and binds thyroid receptors, but blocks them instead of activating them. Where T3 is described as a metabolic accelerator, rT3 is described as a metabolic brake, slowing down the metabolism.

Best Test for Hashimoto's

In most cases of Hashimoto's thyroiditis, blood tests will reveal one or two types of anti-thyroid antibodies. Thyroid peroxidase antibody (TPOAb) is the most common antibody present, and often antibodies against thyroglobulin (TGAb) are found as well. These antibodies may appear decades before a change in TSH is detected.

Thus, TPO antibody screening is always crucial in suspected thyroid disease.

RECOMMENDED THYROID FUNCTION TESTS

☐ TSH
☐ TPO Antibodies
☐ Thyroglobulin Antibodies
☐ Free T4
☐ Free T3
☐ Reverse T3 (Optional)

Misdiagnosis

As many thyroid symptoms are very non-specific, they are often disregarded by the medical community in the initial stages. Patients are dismissed with having depression, stress or anxiety. Thyroid patients are prescribed anti-depressants or anti-anxiety medications without consideration of thyroid function.

Medical studies have shown that up to one-third of people who fail antidepressants report feeling better once started on Cytomel® (a T3, thyroid hormone).[11] Some patients have even been hospitalized and misdiagnosed as having bipolar disorder or schizophrenia when in fact they were suffering from thyroid imbalances.

Additionally, people with bipolar disorder as well as depressive and anxiety disorders were found to have a higher prevalence of anti-thyroid antibodies.[7] To further complicate the issue, lithium, a medication used for bipolar disorder can trigger Hashimoto's. [10]

High titer of TPO antibodies has been associated with distress, obsessive-compulsive symptoms and anxiety.[4] This is likely as a result of increased amount of thyroid hormone being rushed into the bloodstream causing a transient hyperthyroidism. Anyone who has experienced symptoms of hyperthyroidism can describe how terrible this feels. People with anxiety, depression or other mood disorders should have their thyroid function checked, especially TPO antibodies. Some individuals with lifelong psychiatric diagnoses have been able to recover after receiving proper thyroid care.[9]

Prognosis

According to most endocrinologists, the progression from euthyroid (normal thyroid hormone levels) to hypothyroidism is irreversible and ends with complete thyroid cell damage, however, it has been reported that thyroid function spontaneously returned to normal in 20% of patients.[1,8]

These individuals will return to normal thyroid function even after thyroid hormone replacement is withdrawn.

Studies show that once the autoimmune attack ceases, the damaged thyroid has the ability to regenerate. Thyroid ultrasounds will show normal thyroid tissue that has regenerated, and the person will no longer test positive for TPO antibodies. [12]

This regeneration may often be missed in adult patients because they are assumed to have hypothyroidism for life and antibodies and ultrasounds are not usually repeated after the initial diagnosis.

In addition to the ultrasound and TPO antibodies, a test can be done by administering TRH (Thyroid Releasing Hormone), which will cause an increase in T3 and T4 if the thyroid has recovered. This test will help determine if the person can be weaned off thyroid medications. [8]

While this information is readily available in the scientific literature, most physicians do not attempt to administer TRH in an effort to see if patients could be weaned off of their thyroid medications.

Conventional medicine has yet to recognize the impact of lifestyle modifications that can slow down, halt or reverse disease progression. These lifestyle interventions will be the focus of the rest of this book.

Chapter Summary

✓ Test thyroid function using TSH, Free T3, Free T4, TPO Antibodies.
✓ Remission is possible with return to normal thyroid function.

My Story

I struggled with chronic fatigue for seven years before I was diagnosed with Hashimoto's. At first I attributed the fatigue to being a student in a challenging doctorate program with an erratic schedule.

But after graduation, when I started to have a more regular lifestyle, I sought out physicians to inquire about my fatigue, and was told that "everything was normal." Most of them suggested that I was depressed. "But I don't feel depressed, I'm happy!" I always replied. "I'm just really tired. I sleep for twelve hours per night." After a few years, I just gave up trying to find a reason and accepted that I needed more rest than everyone else I knew.

A few years later, new symptoms started emerging gradually, including anxiety, acid reflux, hair loss, and cold intolerance. I slept under two blankets in Southern California.

I had a physical where my TSH was 4.5 µIU/ml (normal 0.4-4.0), however the physician told me: "Your thyroid function is normal. No need to do anything else." He did not test me for antibodies.

The following year I came back again for another physical, and this time my TSH was 8 µIU, and only at that time did the physician recommend consulting an endocrinologist for my thyroid function.

Meanwhile, I had been experiencing symptoms of hypothyroidism for seven years!

"Every great journey begins with a single step"-
Chinese Proverb

3: RESTORING THYROID HORMONE LEVELS

Conventional medicine focuses on restoring normal thyroid function
through the use of supplemental hormones. If we are to use the
analogy of a cup with a hole in it that is leaking liquid to symbolize
the depletion of thyroid hormones, conventional medicine does not
consider the source of the leak (autoimmune destruction), simply, it
keeps adding more water into the cup.

While medication does not address the root cause, it is a crucial first
step to feeling better and reversing the negative effects of
hypothyroidism on the body. Whether one should start replacement
thyroid hormone is primarily determined by lab tests and secondly,
the patient's symptoms, according to conventional guidelines.

Traditionally, physicians did not prescribe thyroid hormones when
someone was considered to have subclinical hypothyroidism
(elevated TSH but normal to borderline low T4 levels), however
some more progressive endocrinologists and physicians are now
recognizing the value of beginning thyroid hormone supplementation
in subclinical hypothyroidism, especially in those who are
experiencing symptoms of hypothyroidism.

Additionally, new guidelines are also recommending to start
supplemental thyroid hormone earlier in the game. Even if T4 levels
are still normal to borderline low. Recommendations are to start
supplemental hormones in subclinical hypothyroidism when the TSH
is above 10 μIU/ml even without any symptoms, and when the TSH
is between 3-10 μIU/ml if symptoms are present.[10, 11]

Hormone supplementation in conventional medicine is considered to
be lifelong, making Hashimoto's a chronic condition that is very
dependent on the traditional medical system with a continued need

for physician visits, lab monitoring and daily medication, with the potential of dose escalation as more thyroid tissue destruction occurs.

Lab tests to repeat thyroid function studies need to be performed four to eight weeks after starting the medication and after any dose changes. Once stable, lab studies should be repeated every six to twelve months, or more frequently in the patient has thyroid symptoms.[4]

Which thyroid medication is best?

Thyroid hormones are known to have a very narrow therapeutic index, they are "Goldilocks" medications, in that have to be dosed just right to ensure effectiveness and prevent adverse drug events. Thyroid hormones are dosed in micrograms, that is just $1/1000^{th}$ of a milligram! When the dose is a teensy bit too high, we may have symptoms of *hyper*thyroidism, and when the dose is a teensy bit too low, we have symptoms of hypothyroidism!

Conventional physicians will usually prescribe Synthroid® or levothyroxine, a synthetic version of T4. Armour® and other animal organ-derived products are not usually recommended by conventional physicians because of past issues with quality control.

In the past, Armour® has had some discrepancies in the dosages between the batches, however, this does not seem to be the case at present time due to improved quality control. Nature-Throid®, another desiccated thyroid medication has never been recalled for inconsistent T4 and T3 hormones. Conventional treatment guidelines state that there is no benefit from taking combination T3/T4 products, and that T4 products are superior, however, most of these claims are based on studies funded by pharmaceutical companies with a vested interest in promoting the use of their own products. [10]

Understanding thyroid physiology, I do believe that combination products may be advantageous for many patients with Hashimoto's.

Some Hashimoto's patients are not able to properly and efficiently convert T4 to T3. For example, zinc is required to convert T4 to T3, and as you will come to learn in the "Depletions & Digestion" chapter, Hashimoto's patients are often deficient in zinc.

Under stressful situations, T4 gets converted to Reverse T3 instead of T3. Reverse T3 is an inactive molecule related to T3 but without any metabolic activity-it is a dud that just takes up space! In the case where a lot of Reverse T3 is produced, adding a combination product that contains T3 will help ensure that the right hormone is getting to the right receptors. Additionally, many patients report that they feel better taking a combination T4/T3 product.

Table 1: Factors that Inhibit T4 to T3 Conversion[9]

Nutrient Depletions	Stress	Aging	Alcohol	Obesity
Chemotherapy	Cigarettes	Diabetes	Fasting	Soy
Medications	Goiterogens	Pesticides	Radiation	Surgery
Kidney and Liver Disease	Heavy Metals	Growth Hormone Deficiency	Low Progesterone	Iodine Excess

National Institute of Health, a government agency (not funded by pharmaceutical grants) conducted a clinical trial to see if desiccated thyroid therapy is advantageous to T4 alone[8]. The authors of the study concluded: "DTE (Desiccated Thyroid Extract) therapy did not result in a significant improvement in quality of life; however, DTE caused modest weight loss and nearly half (48.6%) of the study patients expressed preference for DTE over l-T4 (Levothyroxine). DTE therapy may be relevant for some hypothyroid patients".[13]

Thyroid hormone therapy should be individualized with the patient in mind. Some people report feeling better on natural desiccated hormone, others on compounded medications, while others may feel better taking Synthroid® or another version of synthetic T4.

Some patients may have ethical objections to using animal-derived products like Armour®. Compounded T4/T3 products offer another alternative. These medications also offer the advantage of being made without fillers such as lactose or gluten, which are present in some thyroid medications and can be problematic for thyroid patients (as you will learn in the "Gut" chapter). However, compounded T4/T3 products need to be prepared by a specially trained compounding pharmacist. These compounds are usually much more expensive and may need to be refrigerated to preserve activity.

Some proponents of natural thyroid medications claim that the desiccated glands of animals may be the best option as they also have trace amounts of T1 and T2, which may have undiscovered biological functions.

In contrast, Dr. Alexander Haskell (author of "Hope for Hashimoto's") and Dr. Mark Starr (author of "Hypothyroidism Type II"), report that for some patients, natural thyroid formulations from animal thyroids, such as Armour®, may be perpetuating the autoimmune attack due to containing thyroglobulin and TPO, and they only recommend compounded and synthetic thyroid medications for people with Hashimoto's. [6,7]

If someone starts feeling worse after initially feeling better on desiccated thyroid or has an increase in TPO antibodies after starting desiccated thyroid, switching to a compounded T4/T3 medication may be helpful. Some thyroid advocates report that increasing the dose of desiccated thyroid to a suppressive level will reduce the effect on antibodies. A suppressive dose essentially puts our own thyroid to sleep, and all of the required hormones are obtained from the medication.

Compounded T4/T3

Thyroid compounds are usually prepared in the same physiological ratio that is found in Armour®, however, physicians can elect to change the amount of T3/T4, as the compounding pharmacists are literally making the medications from scratch.

An additional benefit of T4/T3 compounds is that they can be made devoid of any fillers that people may not tolerate, and they do not increase autoimmunity. Most T4/T3 compounds are immediate release versions, like Armour®, however, compounding pharmacists can also make sustained release versions. Some professionals recommend sustained release formulations so that the hormone is released continuously throughout the day, however, these types of formulations may not be absorbed properly by people with Hashimoto's and gut issues.

The downside of T4/T3 compounds is that specially trained compounding pharmacists need to make them, and do take some time to prepare. Additionally, not all compounding pharmacies are equal, and a specialized process is required to prepare an accurate dose of compounded thyroid medications. Thus, patients might have to travel out of their way to find a compounding pharmacy.

Questions to ask your compounding pharmacist:

- ✓ What types of fillers are used?
- ✓ What is the source of the materials?
- ✓ Is the compound slow release or immediate release?

Other Hypoallergenic Options

Nature-Throid®, Westhroid-P® and Tirosint® are other hypoallergenic options. There are many options for thyroid hormone treatment. Each person should work with an open-minded physician to find the thyroid medication that works best for him/her.

Table 2: Thyroid Medications[1,2,4]

Brand Name (Generic Name)	Description
Armour® Thyroid Nature-Throid® Westhroid-P® NP Thyroid® (Thyroid USP):	Desiccated pork thyroid gland T4/T3 combination Mimics the biological ratio of 80% T4 to 20% of T3. T4:T3 ratio of 4:1 May also contain TPO and Thyroglobulin which may perpetuate the autoimmune attack in some
Proloid®: (Thyroglobulin)	Partially purified pork thyroglobulin Gives T4:T3 ratio of 2.5:1
Synthroid®: Synthroid®, Levothyroid®, Levoxyl®, Thyro-Tabs®, Unithroid®(Levothyroxine)	Synthetic T4 Variable absorption among products. Should not switch back and forth between brand/generics.
Cytomel® (Liothyronine)	Synthetic T3
Liotrix® (Thyrolar)	Synthetic T4:T3 in 4:1 ratio (on long-term backorder at the time of writing this book; www.thyrolar.com)
Compounded Thyroid	Tailored dosage forms with unique ratio of T4/T3 and free of allergenic fillers may be prepared by specialized compounding pharmacists. May be formulated as immediate release or slow release. Slow release products may be more difficult to absorb.
Tirosint®	New liquid gelcap formulation of T4, contains only glycerin, gelatin, and water.

Goals of Medication Therapy

The goals of medication therapy are to relieve symptoms and to get the TSH, Free T4, and Free T3 in the normal range. Most endocrinologists consider "normal" TSH to be simply within the reference range, however many patients report "feeling like sloths" with a "normal" TSH of 2.5 µIU/L! Some may need to increase the dose until the TSH is at or below 1 µIU/L.

Thyroid medications that contain T3 such as Armour®, compounded T3/T4, Thyrolar®, and Cytomel® can skew thyroid function test results. When testing thyroid functions, tests should be done before the daily dose of medication is taken. As these medications are generally taken in the morning, the person will want to postpone the medication on test day until after the blood test has been done.

Dosing

Usually the person is started on a low-dose thyroid medication and the dose is increased gradually to normalize TSH, Free T4, and Free T3. This is to avoid a shock to the body of a huge, dramatic change and to determine the appropriate amount needed. After the initial starting dose, the TSH and Free T4/T3 are measured again in four to six weeks to see if they have improved. If the lab ranges are still not at goal, the dose is increased, and labs repeated.

Synthroid® (Levothyroxine): 1.7 mcg/kg daily, and the dose is increased by 25 mcg every four to six weeks.

Armour®, Compounded T3/T4: Start at 30 mg; increase by 15 mg every six weeks.

Nature-Throid®: Start at 32.5mg, increase by 16.25mg every 6 weeks.

Changing Between Thyroid Medications

While dose conversions from Armour® to compounded T3/T4 may be 1:1, there may still be some discrepancies in the dose you receive, so it is important to monitor your symptoms and repeat your labs four to six weeks after switching the thyroid medication to make sure your body is adjusting well.

Table 3: Thyroid Medication Dose Conversions[1,2,4]

Medication Name	Armour®, Compounded T4/T3,	Nature-Throid®	Cytomel®	Synthroid® (levothyroxine)
Equivalent Dose	¼ grain (15 mg)	¼ grain (16.25 mg)		25 mcg
Equivalent Dose	½ grain (30 mg)	½ grain (32.5 mg)	12.5 mcg	50 mcg (0.05 mg)
Equivalent Dose	1 grain (60 mg)	1 grain (65 mg)	25 mcg	100 mcg (0.1 mg)
Equivalent Dose	1 ½ grains (90 mg)	1 ½ grains (97.5 mg)	37.5 mcg	150 mcg (0.15 mg)
Equivalent Dose	2 grains (120 mg)	2 grains (130 mg)	50 mcg	200 mcg (0.2mg)
Equivalent Dose	3 grains (180 mg)	3 grains (195 mg)	75 mcg	300 mcg (0.3 mg)

Other Conventional Treatments

Steroids have been used to suppress the immune process, but antibodies and thyroid dysfunction returned after discontinuation. Chloroquine, an antimalarial drug that is also used for rheumatoid arthritis and cancer, has been shown to reduce anti-thyroid antibodies. Its use is not recommended because of toxic effects.

For cases when the thyroid gland is extremely painful, surgery may be considered. This surgery removes the entire thyroid gland and the person is put on lifelong thyroid replacement hormone.[3,4]

Are Medications Lifelong?

I would like to start off by saying that medications are a great tool in the arsenal that we have to overcome Hashimoto's, and that they are of tremendous benefit while we fix the issues that are contributing to our autoimmune thyroiditis.

Despite the 20% spontaneous recovery rate, most physicians will tell their patients that the supplementation is lifelong. Perhaps it is easier and less expensive to have someone on lifelong pills instead of running tests and attempting to taper down a medication. In some cases a person might become hyperthyroid, which will necessitate a medication dose reduction. In other cases where the medication gets built into our physiology due to hormonal feedback, internal hormone synthesis turns off because there is enough supplemental hormone circulating, and a TRH (Thyroid Releasing Hormone) test needs to be done to see if the thyroid function has recovered.

Lifestyle interventions can also help with reducing TPO antibodies, reversing hypothyroidism and Hashimoto's, preventing other diseases, and will make most people feel better. Some people might be able to reduce and eliminate the need for thyroid medications when the autoimmune attack ceases and the thyroid gland is able to regenerate.

Medications versus Lifestyle Interventions

For those already taking thyroid supplements, it is crucial never to stop the medication abruptly. Abrupt cessation can lead to severe hypothyroid symptoms and cause a rapid escalation of TSH, leading to more thyroid damage. Gradual tapering of the medication is necessary and should only be done under the supervision of a physician.

I know some people refuse to take thyroid medications, and feel that taking thyroid medications is like giving up! But that is not the case! Think of medications as one tool in your toolbox for overcoming Hashimoto's. We can use medications to help us feel better while we work everything else out.

Do not think of medications as a life sentence, in many cases, especially if the condition was caught early, you may be able to get off them once you fix the "leaks" in your body that are contributing to the autoimmune destruction of the thyroid. However, if your TSH is elevated for a prolonged period of time, this could be very harmful to the rest of your body and hinder your recovery.

Bottom line, if you have an elevated TSH and/or have thyroid symptoms, you will likely benefit from thyroid medications. There is no need for you to suffer while you search for the root cause of your condition. Optimizing medication is the first step for feeling well with Hashimoto's.

Chapter Summary

- ✓ Discuss starting or changing thyroid medication with your doctor if having low thyroid symptoms.
- ✓ Combination T3/T4 medications may be helpful for many.
- ✓ Retest TPO antibodies after starting natural desiccated thyroid.

"Autoimmune disease: because the only thing tough enough to kick my a** is me"-Unknown

4: WHAT IS AN AUTOIMMUNE CONDITION?

In simple terms, autoimmunity means that a person's own immune system mistakenly recognizes normally occurring physiological processes as foreign invaders and attacks itself. Hashimoto's Thyroiditis is the first autoimmune condition recognized in medicine. You may have heard hypothyroidism described as having a "sluggish" or "underactive" thyroid. This is something that is thought to happen with advanced age, but this is not the case with the thyroid in autoimmune hypothyroidism. The thyroid is working overtime to produce adequate hormone while the immune system gradually destroys it. The problem is not with the thyroid's performance, rather with the immune system's performance.

Basically, the theory goes like this:

1) Thyroid cells are damaged by a trigger, such as iodine, fluoride, viral infection, etc.
2) Dying thyroid cells send out a stress signal.
3) Immune cells come in to "save" the thyroid from attackers.
4) Immune cells attack thyroid instead.
5) More thyroid cell damage occurs.
6) Body runs out of resources to regenerate thyroid cells.
7) Thyroid is no longer able to produce enough hormone.

Perfect Storm

There is not just one event that causes the autoimmunity, but instead, a series of events has to line up just right to create the perfect storm, or perfect circumstances, for developing autoimmunity.

Recent exciting advances in autoimmunity have been made by world-renowned celiac disease researcher and gastroenterologist Alessio Fasano. Dr. Fasano and his colleagues have suggested that there are three factors that need to be present for autoimmunity to develop:

1) Genetic predisposition
2) Exposure to antigen (trigger)
3) Intestinal permeability

The intestinal permeability and triggers cause an immune system imbalance that results in the body no longer recognizing itself from a foreign invader. [1,2]

How is increased intestinal permeability connected to autoimmune disorders?

Your intestinal tract has the surface area of a tennis court and has the largest concentration of immune cells, as well as the same number of neurons as your spinal cord.

Researchers have found that in addition to digesting and absorbing nutrients, the intestine is also responsible for keeping the potentially harmful substances from our environment out of our bodies. The intestinal wall, in particular, has recently been credited for keeping the body from recognizing itself versus foreign antigens.

When the intestinal wall becomes more permeable, the body loses its ability to recognize benign substances, such as our own cells and foods we eat, and instead treats them as though they were foreign invaders such as bacteria and viruses.

Zonulin is a recently discovered human protein that reversibly increases intestinal permeability. This protein is measured in excessive amounts in individuals with autoimmune conditions such as rheumatoid arthritis, Hashimoto's, multiple sclerosis, type 1 diabetes, and celiac disease (see the "Gut" chapter for more details). [1,2]

How do triggers work?

Let's use iodine as our sample trigger.

When iodine enters the cell, TPO, the enzyme that oxidizes iodide to the reactive iodine is released to allow the iodine to attach to tyrosine residues in thyroglobulin to form thyroid hormones. (Refer to Chapter 2 for more details).[3]

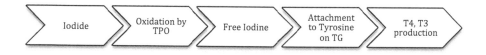

In normal thyroid cells, the antioxidant glutathione peroxidase neutralizes the hydrogen peroxide, preventing thyroid cell damage. This antioxidant is made from glutathione and selenium. Depletions, including selenium and glutathione deficiency, have been recognized as a trigger for Hashimoto's.

The following mechanism explains why supplementing with iodide can cause an immune system flare-up:

1) Iodide gets in the blood.
2) Iodide gets oxidized to Iodine by TPO.
3) Oxygen-free radicals are formed during oxidation.
4) In the absence of selenium, free radicals cause damage to the thyroid cells instead of being neutralized.
5) Lymphocytes (white blood cells) infiltrate the thyroid tissue to repair the damage and produce inflammation of the thyroid.
6) Inflammation causes further destruction of thyroid tissues.
7) More white blood cells infiltrate the thyroid.

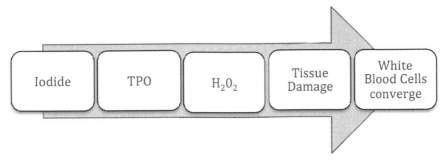

Figure 2: Iodine as a Trigger

Our immune system evolved to protect us from harmful foreign invaders. As TPO expression results in oxidative damage, our immune system starts recognizing it as an enemy. Whenever the immune system recognizes a foreign invader, it also will form antibodies against the invader. In the case of Hashimoto's, the target is the TPO enzyme.

Thyroid peroxidase antibodies (TPOAb) are formed in response to this thyroid injury. These antibodies activate the immune system, which leads to an all-out search and destroy mission on the enemy.

The immune system then launches an attack to try to clear the body of the invader, unfortunately, in this case, the immune cells target healthy thyroid tissue instead.

Hashimoto's has been classified as a Type IV hypersensitivity, which is called a delayed type hypersensitivity ("self-allergy"). Unlike the other types of immune reactions, the damage to the thyroid tissue is not antibody mediated, but rather the antibodies "mark" the thyroid cells, and the attack is done by antigen-specific cytotoxic T-lymphocytes (lymph cells) that attack the thyroid cells. [5, 6]

Lymphocytes (also known as white blood cells) begin to enter the thyroid and begin to destroy it, causing scarring, which leads to a decreased ability to produce thyroid hormones.

The production of TPO antibodies will perpetuate the attack on the thyroid whenever TPO is expressed. These antibodies will keep forming as long as TPO is around, and this will eventually lead to so much scarring to the thyroid tissues that the thyroid will no longer be able to produce adequate hormone. More than 90% of people with Hashimoto's have thyroid peroxidase antibodies (TPOAb). [6]

Additionally, antibodies may also be formed to thyroglobulin (Tg), the protein that is an intermediary in the thyroid hormone production pathway. Iodine attaches to tyrosine residues in thyroglobulin, forming a new molecule. In the presence of iodine, thyroglobulin becomes more visible to the immune system, it has even been suggested that excess iodine may create "mutant" thyroglobulin molecules that may be especially targeted by immune cells. Thyroglobulin also acts as a storage molecule for thyroid hormones, so iodine consumption may actually trigger a thyrotoxic episode of hyperthyroidism that can cause palpitations, anxiety, and agitation due to destruction of the storage protein and spillover of the stored thyroid hormones. About 80% of people with Hashimoto's have thyroglobulin antibodies (TgAb). [6]

Collectively, all antibodies directed against thyroid processes are known as microsomal antibodies, however, this term is sometimes used to refer to TPOAb specifically when discussing different types of antibodies. They are classified as Immunoglobulin G (IgG) types of antibodies that are also responsible for fighting infections as well as delayed types of food sensitivities.

Initially, the production of self-reactive and autoantibodies occurs in the draining lymph nodes but may then move over to the thyroid.

In the case of Hashimoto's; antibodies are produced to thyroid peroxidase enzyme or to thyroglobulin. Most people with Hashimoto's will have an elevation of one or both of these antibodies, indicating an active immune system attack.

Antibodies are used as an indicator of autoimmune activity—the more antibodies, the more thyroid damage is occurring. Various labs use different ranges for antibodies. Generally, having TPO antibodies above 30 kU/L is consistent with having Hashimoto's. Antibodies above 500 kU/L are considered aggressive, while antibodies of less than 100 kU/L are associated with a reduced risk of progressing to hypothyroidism.

Taking iodine with elevated TPO antibodies has been described as "pouring more gas on the fire," as it flares up Hashimoto's and causes an increase in antibodies. Most integrative Hashimoto's professionals recommend avoiding or limiting iodine until the TPO antibodies are no longer elevated, or until they are below 100 kU/L.

Reducing Autoimmunity

It was once believed that once the autoimmune process is activated, it becomes independent of continuous exposure to the environmental trigger and becomes self-sustaining and irreversible.

However, examples of autoimmunity have discredited the "irreversible" aspect of this theory. It has been shown that continuous environmental triggers are necessary to perpetuate the process. This means that the autoimmune process can be stopped and reversed when the triggers are eliminated. One example of this is celiac disease, an autoimmune condition where gluten, an environmental trigger, has been identified. In most cases of classical celiac disease, all symptoms resolve when the environmental trigger (gluten) is removed.

Table 4: Thyroid Events Amsterdam (THEA) Score[4]

The THEA score is used to help estimate the risk of developing hypothyroidism within five years in people who have TPO antibodies and relatives of those with thyroid diseases. Note: Higher antibodies are associated with a greater risk of developing hypothyroidism.

Characteristic	Hypothyroid Event
TSH, mIU/L	
<0.4	0
0.4-2.0	0
>2.0-4.0	3
>4.0-5.7	6
>5.7	9
TPO Antibodies, kU/L	
≤ 100	0
>100-1000	3
>1000-10,000	6
>10,000	9
Family Background	
2 Relatives with Graves'	0
2 Relatives with Hashimoto's	3
Maximum THEA Score	21

Score Interpretation

Score	Risk Category	Percent hypothyroid within five years
0-7	Low	1.6%
8-10	Medium	12.2%
11-15	High	30.8%
16-21	Very High	85.7%

Adapted from Strieder TGA, Tijssen JGP, Wenzel BE, Endert E, Wiersinga WM. Prediction of Progression to Overt Hypothyroidism or Hyperthyroidism in female relatives of patients with autoimmune thyroid diseases using the Thyroid Events Amsterdam (THEA) Score. Arch Intern Med/Vol 168 (No 15), Aug 11/25, 2008

Antibody Memory

IgG subclass antibodies have a half-life of 21 days, and stick around on immune cells for about two to three months. They need constant "reminders" in the form of an antigen so that their production continues. If the antigen is removed, the antibodies will go away as well. The time period required for them to completely forget about the antigen and disappear is nine to twelve months. [5]

The following things need to be in place for the antibodies to forget about the thyroid:

1) The thyroid stops expressing TPO.
2) The thyroid cells are not damaged and able to regenerate.
3) There are no substances that look like TPO (glandulars, gluten, infections, other triggers).
4) The immune system is balanced.
5) The autoimmune cells are confused by a decoy.

Some of these requirements are quick and easy, and others will take some time ...

The thyroid will stop expressing TPO for two reasons. One of them is thyroid destruction, which we do not want; the other is thyroid suppression. Thyroid suppression is induced by limiting iodine and taking a thyroid supplement to bring TSH to 1 mIU/L or so. This can take up to three months.

In the case of autoimmune conditions, traditional and alternative medicine practitioners may focus on rebalancing the immune system (i.e., steroids and immune-modulating drugs used in traditional medicine; herbs, supplements, or acupuncture used in alternative medicine).

While this approach may be helpful for taming the immune system in the short term or overcoming autoimmune flares, it is often a temporary solution and the immune system may become imbalanced again once the medications, acupuncture, and herbs and supplements are stopped if the underlying issue that lead to the immune system imbalance is not addressed. Thus we can say that immune modulation treats only the symptoms, and not the root cause.

As we can't change genes, our approach to addressing the root cause of Hashimoto's is threefold:

1) Reducing triggers
2) Eliminating intestinal permeability
3) Providing the body with nutrients to regenerate

Eliminating and identifying triggers and toxins will likely take a few weeks to a few months. Providing the thyroid with the nutrition needed to help rebuild and detoxify will likely take three to six months.

Rebalancing the immune system by addressing the root cause of autoimmunity (intestinal permeability, gut dysbiosis, infections) may take one to three years, but in the meantime, we can modulate the immune system and throw our thyroid antibodies a decoy.

Thytrophin PMG: Decoy

Thytrophin PMG is a supplement that can be helpful in neutralizing the circulating antibodies to TPO and thyroglobulin. In Hashimoto's, white blood cells are attracted to the thyroid as a result of a stress signal that is given off by dying thyroid cells.

Thytrophin PMG is a bovine thyroid extract of the stress signal and confuses the antibodies and white blood cells. Instead of attacking the thyroid tissues, the antibodies attach to the PMG extract. This gives the thyroid a break from attack, allowing it to regenerate. Thytrophin PMG does not contain TPO or thyroglobulin like many glandular products and thus it does not induce an autoimmune reaction against the thyroid gland.[7]

This supplement is another tool that can be used to help recover thyroid function while working toward finding and treating the root cause of Hashimoto's and associated triggers.

Antibody testing following the initiation of this supplement is recommended.

Chapter Summary

✓ Hashimoto's is an autoimmune condition with antibodies directed against the thyroid.
✓ The perfect storm of genes, triggers, and intestinal permeability must all be present to cause Hashimoto's.
✓ Immune modulation is only a temporary solution.
✓ The approach to overcoming Hashimoto's is threefold: removing triggers, reducing intestinal permeability and nourishing the thyroid and can take three months to three years.
✓ Thytrophin PMG can act as a decoy for thyroid antibodies while we work to fix the root cause.

PART II: FINDING YOUR ROOT CAUSE

"Whether you think you can or can't you are right."-Henry Ford

5: FINDING YOUR ROOT CAUSE

I wrote this book to guide others with Hashimoto's to find and treat the root cause of their own condition, based on the research I did to overcome my own condition. I am a firm believer in patient empowerment and self-management, and what I love the most about being a medical professional is the opportunity to teach others how to take care of themselves and their loved ones.

While you may need to utilize the services of various health-care professionals throughout your healing journey, the push to get better and to keep asking questions has to come from you. After all, you know yourself better than anyone else.

Additionally, while there are some health-care professionals who are very knowledgeable about treating Hashimoto's, after reading this book, you will likely know more about your condition than most of them. I hope that this information will empower you to be at the center of your own care team!

Some medical professionals will say that it is impossible to return to normal thyroid function after Hashimoto's, but that is not true. They just don't know how to get there. People are recovering from Hashimoto's every day. Some of them are recovering by accident, and some on purpose.

This book will give you the tools to find and treat the root cause of Hashimoto's so that you too can get better—on purpose!

What's Really Going on in Hashimoto's?

Hashimoto's is a complicated condition with many layers that need to be unraveled. While conventional medicine only looks at each body system as a separate category, and is only concerned with the thyroid's ability to produce thyroid hormone, Hashimoto's is more than just hypothyroidism.

Our thyroid is part of a complicated body system and does not live by itself in a vacuum.

Often patients with Hashimoto's will present with acid reflux, nutrient deficiencies, anemia, increased intestinal permeability, food sensitivities, gum disorders, and hypoglycemia, in addition to "typical" hypothyroid symptoms that were discussed in Chapter 2.

The body becomes stuck in a chronic state of immune system overload, adrenal insufficiency, gut dysbiosis, impaired digestion, inflammation, and thyroid hormone release abnormalities.

These changes can lead to symptoms of anxiety, depression and chronic fatigue that are often seen with Hashimoto's.

This cycle is interrelated and reinforces itself through a positive feedback loop, meaning the cycle is self sustaining and will continue causing more and more symptoms until an external factor intervenes and breaks the cycle apart.

Unfortunately, simply adding thyroid supplement to the mix will not result in full recovery for most thyroid patients. Additionally, supporting just the thyroid may weaken the adrenals and immune balance, which will in turn perpetuate the vicious cycle. Thus each intervention needs to be counterbalanced to ensure that we are not inadvertently causing an imbalance in another part of our body.

The lifestyle interventions discussed in this book aim to dismantle the vicious cycle piece by piece. We start with the simplest modifications, by removing triggers, and follow with repairing the other broken systems to restore equilibrium, allowing the body to heal itself.

Figure 3: Hashimoto's Thyroiditis: Vicious Cycle

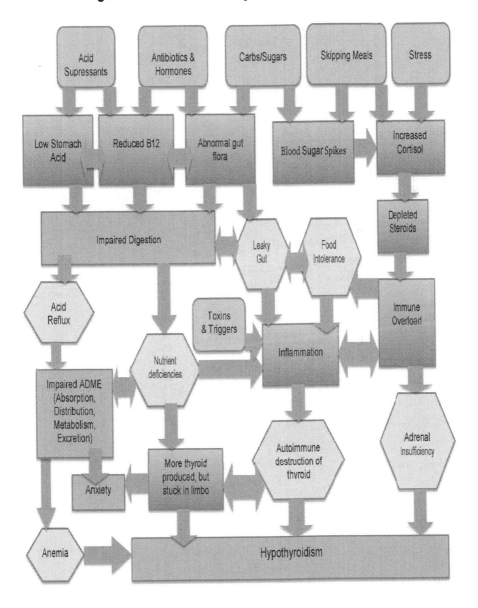

Hashimoto's is a complex chain of events that reinforces itself through a feedback loop. This vicious cycle will continue in the direction of its momentum until an external factor intervenes and breaks the cycle.

Image by: Izabella Wentz, PharmD, FASCP

How To Find Your Path

"Every strike brings me closer to a home run."-Babe Ruth

Healing from any chronic condition and moving towards better health is a journey. You may stumble before you succeed. I know that I struggled for a few years before I finally found what worked for me.

Don't Give Up, Dig At It!

How do you find the root cause of your thyroid condition? You have to DIG AT IT. Once you do, you will know what types of changes you need to implement to make yourself feel better.

The acronym **DIG AT IT** stands for the following:

Depletions, Digestion
Iodine, Inflammation, Infection, Immune Imbalance
Gut, Gluten

Adrenals, Alkaline Phosphatase
Triggers

Intolerances
Toxins

As you read each chapter dedicated to the above-mentioned headings, pay special attention to the quizzes and assessments to determine which types of risk factors you may have had for developing Hashimoto's.

You will then create your own Health Timeline. This timeline should include an overall health history as far back as you can remember. Infections, periods of severe stress, the use of medications (especially antibiotics, antacids, and oral contraceptives), accidents, and exposure to toxins should be especially noted.

Underline the events that may have contributed to your illness.

After you have completed your timeline, you will be ready for the "How to Heal" phase of the book which includes the "Getting Better", "Diet", "Supplements" and "Testing" chapters.

I am providing a sample Health Timeline for your reference in the Appendix.

Additionally, as you start to make interventions, you should keep a journal of how various lifestyle choices impact your wellbeing. It may be helpful to keep a simple running tally with the following headings:

1. Things that make me better
2. Things that make me worse

This will enable you to tailor the healing plan to your own needs and individuality.

This book is divided by various body organs for the sake of keeping things organized and to avoid overwhelming the reader with too much physiology and biology all at once, but it's really important to keep the big picture in mind. Our body is a complete system—we can't isolate one body part without affecting another.

Chapter Summary

✓ DIG AT IT to find and treat the root cause of Hashimoto's.

"Bad digestion is the root of all evil"-
Hippocrates

6: DIGESTION & DEPLETIONS

We have learned that in the case of Hashimoto's, as with all cases of autoimmune conditions, the problem is with the immune system, and not the particular organ that is attacked, such as the thyroid.

In fact, in most cases of Hashimoto's, the thyroid is working overtime to keep up thyroid hormone production despite being attacked by the immune system.

Autoimmunity may be in part triggered by nutrient depletions, while nutrient depletions may also result from the increased thyroid cell turnover.

As a word of caution, most "Thyroid Support" formulas promoted by alternative medicine practitioners that promise to restore a "sluggish thyroid" will not correct an autoimmune thyroid condition, and depending on the active ingredients, may actually worsen the condition.

Some nutrients are essential to thyroid function, while others are required for proper immune system, liver, gut, and adrenal function, and a depletion thus may be compromising thyroid function directly or indirectly.

In contrast, an excess of other nutrients may be perpetuating an autoimmune thyroid.

Smart nutrient supplementation can be helpful with not only improving thyroid function, but also reducing TPO antibodies.

The following helpful lifestyle interventions will be discussed in further detail in this chapter:

- Causes of depletions
- Impact of thyroid hormones on digestion
- Addressing depletions
- Selenium
- N-Acetyl Cysteine (glutathione precursor)

CAUSES OF DEPLETIONS

Why Do We Have Nutrient Depletions?

Various substances present in our comfort-craving, health-compromising American lifestyle can have a profound impact on our nutrient levels.

Conventional versus Organic Farming

Conventional commercial farming practices reduce our nutrient content as vegetables and fruit absorb their nutrients from the soil in which they are grown.

Conventional crops are grown with synthetic fertilizers, synthetic pesticides, and are in the same fields over and over again, causing soils to become depleted. If you live in the Midwest you will drive past cornfields that have been in the same place for decades.

Fruit and vegetables are picked before they are ripe enough in order to survive transport across the country. This does not allow them to continue getting their nutrients from an already depleted soil.

In contrast, organic farmers rotate their crops, fertilize their soils with natural fertilizers such as compost, and rely on nature's pesticides by encouraging insect predators to make the farms their home. Organic farmers also make sure to pick vegetables when they are ripe, and these vegetables have been found to be much more rich in nutrients. One study found that some organic vegetables had almost 90% more nutrients compared with their conventionally grown counterparts.

Food Processing

The way our food is processed also takes out many of the nutrients normally present. Let's take wheat, for example. Wheat starts off as a wheat kernel that is made up of starch, nutrient-filled bran and germ. The bran and germ are removed, leaving behind just the starch, a.k.a. "flour." This flour is then bleached so that it is more aesthetically pleasing. A couple of synthetic B vitamins, iron, and folic acid are added in.

Found in bread, cereal, waffles, wraps, sandwiches, pasta, crackers, and most processed foods, processed wheat products are the foundation of the standard American diet and yet they are devoid of nutrients.

Every time someone consumes these products, they actually cause the body to lose nutrients instead of gain them!

If that wasn't bad enough, wheat products also contain gluten, a protein that is toxic to many individuals, and has been connected to many autoimmune conditions, especially Hashimoto's.

The Folly of Convenience

Conventional foods found in the Standard American Diet (SAD), devoid of nutrients and full of empty calories, lead us to be nutrient deficient.

Additionally, high-carbohydrate diets, oral contraceptives, antibiotics, and acid-suppressing medications also shift the type of intestinal bacteria we have in our intestinal tracts. These bacteria are responsible for extracting vitamins from our foods as well as keeping peace within our guts. (More about this in the "Immune Imbalance" and "Gut" chapters).

Do You Like Tomatoes?

Commercial growers pick tomatoes when they are green and spray them with ethylene gas (a hormone that accelerates ripening) before they send them to the various stores where they will be sold. This leads to the tomatoes all looking very pretty and red, but tasting like, let's face it, rubbery slush.

Growing up in Poland, where organic farming was very prevalent, I only ate organic tomatoes from my grandmother's garden. My mother continued the tradition when we came to the United States and started growing her own tomatoes in our small backyard outside of Chicago.

I remember how surprised my American friends were when they saw me eating tomatoes "like an apple." "How can you eat tomatoes like that?" They were shocked! But as soon as they tried one of my mother's homegrown heirloom tomatoes, they understood. If you think you don't like tomatoes, try an heirloom tomato from your local farmers' market.

MEDICATIONS AND DEPLETIONS

Acid-Suppressing Medications[3,4]

Drug Category	Nutrient Depletions
Gastric Acid Reducers:	Beneficial flora
	Beta carotene
Proton Pump Inhibitors (PPIs),	Boron
Common names: pantoprazole,	Calcium
Aciphex®, Prilosec®, Nexium®	Chromium
	Copper
H2 Receptor Antagonists	Digestive acids
Common names: famotidine,	Folic acid
Pepcid®	Iron
	Phosphorus
	Selenium
	Thiamin
	Vitamin B_{12}
	Vitamin C
	Vitamin D
	Vitamin E
	Vitamin K
	Zinc

Just about everyone knows someone who has acid reflux. This condition is also very common among those with Hashimoto's.

Why? Processed wheat products, pasteurized dairy products devoid of natural enzymes, and more junk, junk, and junk that we are shoving in our mouths day in and day out. Our digestive systems are trying to tell us something: "Stop feeding me this junk, give me something real."

But what does our modern society do to our bodies instead? It gives them a pill, to shut them up. Billions of dollars are spent on over-the-counter antacids, as well prescription acid-suppressing medications. In 2010, Proton Pump Inhibitors, acid-suppressing medications such as Nexium®, Prilosec®, and Prevacid®, were the third-highest selling class of drug in the United States, accounting for $13.9 billion in annual sales.

As the name would imply, acid-suppressing medications suppress our stomach's acid production. But stomach acid is necessary for breaking down foods, especially proteins.

I consider acid reflux, in most cases, to be a sign that you are not feeding your body adequately. Perhaps you are eating a food that is causing you inflammation (please see the "Intolerances" chapter for more information).

The reality is, most people with "acid reflux" have low acid, not high acid. Depletion in the vitamin B_{12} is often responsible for inadequate acid production. Furthermore, suppressing stomach acid prevents us from extracting iron and vitamin B_{12} from foods, resulting in yet another vicious cycle and leading to other digestive problems, anemia, hair loss, and even neurological problems.

Practices in the use of Proton Pump Inhibitors and other acid-suppressing medications have recently come under FDA scrutiny because of increased risks of bone fractures and questionable need.

Most people should not use Proton Pump Inhibitors (PPIs) for extended periods of time. Of course, there may be legitimate reasons one might need to take a medication to suppress acid, such as in the treatment of a bleeding peptic ulcer in the hospital. However, the consensus seems to be that PPIs are overused and overprescribed for GERD (gastroesophageal reflux disease), the most common reason for prescribing these medications. If you are willing to give up the convenience of taking a pill so you can "eat whatever you want," and explore the reason you are actually experiencing these symptoms, your overall health will greatly improve.

Note for coming off from PPIs: These medications will cause an acid rebound if they are discontinued suddenly. A gradual tapering of the medication is recommended while you explore alternatives. For example, if you have been taking two tablets daily, go to one per day for one week, then every other day.

You can also make the transition to Pepcid® (famotidine) an over-the-counter medication as you begin to get off the PPI. Pepcid is a different kind of acid blocker that does not cause rebound. While it is preferred to the PPI, it is still not appropriate for long term use for GERD. You will then taper off the Pepcid® after a week or two as you explore your diet.

Yogi's Ginger Tea is helpful for acid reflux and can help in the transition process.

Got reflux?

My story from the www.thyroidrootcause.org blog

I did too. It started with a chronic cough, pain, burning, and a choking sensation...I tried every over the counter product possible...I saw my primary care doctor, an allergist, a gastroenterologist, an Ear Nose and Throat doctor, and finally had a barium swallow test swallowing a nasty chalky substances... The test showed I had a sliding hiatal hernia with spontaneous reflux.

I drank gallons of milk trying to soothe the burn. I drank bottles of Mylanta®, and always had a bottle of antacids nearby. I tried

Nexium®, Prilosec®, Aciphex®, Pepcid® and even considered surgery. The acid reflux persisted.

For three freaking years I slept nearly upright. For three years I avoided red wine, tomato sauces, oranges and all of the other "acidic" foods I was told to avoid. The acid reflux continued.

I didn't give up the fight...I went the holistic route...tried to get adjustments from a chiropractor to push my hiatal hernia back in. Tried yoga to relax more. Tried ginger tea. Cut out caffeine. Took more magnesium. The acid reflux didn't give...

And then, just when I nearly gave up and thought I would just have to live with it...I made one change to my diet that I thought would never ever make any sort of difference, and there it was, completely gone forever within **3 DAYS** of making this change, after **3 YEARS** of almost daily suffering, my chronic cough was gone and has never come back!

So what was that change? I cut out dairy. I had been eating it my whole life without any apparent problems so I would have never suspected it would be the culprit of my digestive troubles. I had an IgA food intolerance test that showed I was sensitive to it.

Since I cut out dairy almost two years ago I haven't had reflux since...(except for the few times I accidentally consumed something that contained dairy).

Will cutting dairy be the change that makes all the difference of you? I don't know.

But don't give up. You may be one small change away from feeling well!

Estrogen/Progesterone Containing Products[3,4]

Drug Category	Nutrient Depletions
Female hormones such as oral contraceptives or hormone replacement therapy Other names: birth control pills, estrogen/progesterone combination pills, estrogens, progesterone Common brand names: Yaz®, Mircette®, Ortho-Tri-Cyclen®, Premarin®	Beneficial flora DHEA Folate Magnesium Melatonin Riboflavin Selenium Thiamin Vitamin A Vitamin B5 (pantothenic acid) Vitamin B6/pyridoxine Vitamin B_{12} Vitamin C/ascorbic acid Zinc

Oral contraceptives, or birth control pills, are a great convenience. We can take one little pill a day, and stop our ovulation. No more worries about getting pregnant. I know that I have relied on birth control pills to help with heavy menstrual bleeding and skipping periods while on vacation. Birth control has helped me pursue my career and passions in my twenties before I was ready to be a mother. But I wish I had known about the risks associated with "the pill," such as the changes in beneficial bacteria and the nutrient depletions that can cause so many health problems. It's possible that birth control pills are one of the reasons that autoimmune conditions are more common in women than in men.

Additionally, I had never been taught about alternatives to birth control pills. I knew that condoms had a pretty high failure rate for most typical users and as far as natural family planning methods, I went by the old joke, "What do you call people who practice the rhythm method?" "Parents."

However, the rhythm method aside, there are reliable methods of natural family planning that are based on women's reproductive cycles.

Please see the "Triggers" chapter on more information about birth control pills as triggers as well as reliable methods of natural family planning.

Antibiotics

Drug Category	Nutrient Depletions
Antibiotics Common names: penicillin, Cipro®, cephalexin, Z-pack®, many others	Beneficial flora B vitamins Calcium Magnesium Iron

I want to preface this section by saying that antibiotic medications are life-savers and a tremendous advancement in modern medicine, and I would never tell someone with a serious acute condition such as a kidney infection, respiratory infection, or abscess to refuse antibiotics. That said, antibiotics are greatly overused and can have many negative health consequences.

Beneficial flora bacteria are primarily divided into two categories: Gram positive (many of the friendly species) and Gram negative (many of the ones that can become toxic in our bodies if too many are present).

Bacterial infections may be either Gram positive or negative, and while some of the newer antibiotics may be more specific to one kind of bacteria, most antibiotics are "broad spectrum," meaning they kill all kinds of bacteria. Most antibiotics do not know the difference between the bad bacteria that are causing your infection, or the good bacteria that are helping you with digestion, vitamin extraction and keeping peace within your intestinal track.

This can lead to an unfair advantage to the opportunistic bacteria and fungi in our bodies, allowing them to take over while our good bacteria are destroyed. Antibiotics can actually kill off our beneficial flora—for example, your dairy loving lactobacilli—and make us unable to digest dairy.

As the beneficial bacteria make up our immune system, antibiotic use is a suspected cause of an increase of allergies, chronic disease, autoimmune conditions, digestive issues, and even cancer.

Most antibiotics, when used for appropriate times in appropriate doses, should not be an issue for people who follow nutrient-dense diets full of beneficial bacteria.

But overuse of antibiotics is a well-documented issue in the U.S. Multiple coalitions exist to try to address overuse and appropriate use of antibiotics for bacterial infections.

For example, many people will see their doctors because of cold or flu symptoms. These infections are usually caused by viral pathogens, but people will still receive amoxicillin or another broad-spectrum antibiotic. These antibiotics will not help with the cold or flu as they do not work against viruses or fungi, only bacteria. Instead, the antibiotics will have a negative impact the beneficial bacteria.

Another example that comes to mind is that of antibiotics which are often prescribed for acne and are continued for many years. Acne can be very difficult for vulnerable and sensitive teenagers to deal with, and many teens report having an increased self-esteem after improving acne, however there are alternatives to antibiotics. As we are now getting to understand that acne is related to bacteria, and we can affect the bacterial presence by our food choices, people should not be surprised to learn that many cases of acne can be improved with a nutrient-rich/junk-free diet.

I would advise parents and teens to try the dietary approach first. Good fats like avocado, green smoothies, and avoidance of allergenic foods like dairy and gluten may be of much help and prevent the need for a prescription.

THYROID FUNCTION AND NUTRIENT EXTRACTION

Hypothyroidism, in itself, will lead to poor extraction of minerals and vitamins from our food sources. Thyroid hormones determine our metabolism throughout the entire body. As such, the digestive tract is not spared, particularly the intestines. Lack of sufficient thyroid hormones makes nutrient extraction more difficult and less efficient, and can in itself lead to nutrient deficiencies.

A lack of thyroid hormone leads to low temperatures that not only make us uncomfortable in breezy situations, but can also have an impact on hormone synthesis and other important body processes such as digestion, hair growth, skin turnover and regeneration, wound healing, etc.

Achlorhydria, constipation, and incomplete digestion of fibrous plant materials have been associated with hypothyroidism.[7]

Most people with thyroid conditions and adrenal fatigue will have no stomach acid, or low stomach acid (hydrochloric acid or HCl), which is necessary to break down protein. This is known as "achlorhydria", or "hypochlorhydria", respectively. The lack of adequate digestive enzymes leads to a depletion of amino acids, iron, B_{12}, zinc and other nutrients obtained from protein. Symptoms include gas, heartburn, bloating, and heaviness in the stomach after eating a protein meal.

Liver function tests may be disturbed in up to 50% of people with hypothyroidism, leading to reduced output of bile, which helps us digest lipids. Notably, bile stones and gallstones are also more common in Hashimoto's. [7]

People with Hashimoto's are also five times more likely to be diagnosed with Celiac disease. Recently, gluten intolerance has been described as a spectrum, with only the most severe cases of damage being diagnosed with Celiac disease. Additionally, some people with Hashimoto's may present with a celiac-like intolerance to milk proteins (whey and/or casein), egg proteins (ovalbumin), or soy proteins.

Many of these cases are undiagnosed, and when people continue to eat these foods, they are damaging their intestines and robbing themselves of vital nutrients. It sounds surprising, but even people who are overweight may be completely malnourished and nutrient depleted because of the foods they eat. Tests for food intolerances are available and will be discussed in the "Intolerances" and "Testing" chapters of this book.

ADDRESSING DEPLETIONS

Low Stomach Acid

The use of digestive enzymes, probiotics, as well as supplemental acid may be needed to help digest protein. Betaine with Pepsin is a supplement used to raise stomach acid levels and is available for purchase in capsule forms.

Dose: Betaine with Pepsin should be taken after a protein-rich meal, starting with one capsule per meal. The dose should be increased by one more capsule at each meal, until symptoms of too much acid are felt (burping, burning, etc.). At that point, you will know that your dose is one capsule less than what resulted in symptoms.

Betaine with Pepsin Titration Example:

Meal No. 1: One capsule, no symptoms

Meal No. 2: Two capsules, no symptoms

Meal No. 3: Three capsules, no symptoms

Meal No. 4: Four capsules. felt slight burning in throat

Correct dose is: Three capsules per meal

Many people will be amazed how much more energy they have after they start taking digestive enzymes with their meals. I know I felt like a brand new person after starting Betaine with Pepsin.

The digestive enzymes should stimulate your body's own production of acid, and help you extract nutrients from your food. Alternatively, lemon juice and apple cider vinegar can also help to produce more digestive acid. After some time, you should be able to get off the enzymes as your own body begins to produce enough digestive acid.. If you find that your stomach acid production does not return on its own, consider testing for H. Pylori (more in "Infections" chapter).

Nutrients Required for Proper Thyroid Function:

Selenium, iron, vitamin A, vitamin E, the B vitamins, potassium iodine, and zinc are all required for proper thyroid function. Other nutrients, although not directly involved in thyroid function, are also essential for proper immune system, gut, liver and adrenal function.

Most people who are diagnosed with Hashimoto's will also present with low levels of vitamin B_{12}, antioxidants selenium, vitamin E and glutathione, as well as zinc and ferritin (the iron storage protein).

B_{12}

Low levels of B_{12} may lead to anemia, underdevelopment of villi and impaired digestion. Vitamin B_{12} from our diet is found in animal proteins. B_{12} is released for absorption by the activity of hydrochloric acid and protease, an enzyme in the stomach. Low levels of hydrochloric acid commonly found in those with Hashimoto's put people at risk for B_{12} deficiency. Intake of breads and cereals fortified with folic acid may mask this deficiency on standard lab tests.

Vitamin B_{12} is naturally found in animal products including fish, meat, poultry, eggs, milk, and milk products. Vitamin B_{12} is generally not present in plant foods, and thus vegetarians and especially vegans are at a greater risk for deficiency.

Using a vitamin B_{12} supplement is essential for vegans, and may be helpful for those with low stomach acid until the condition is corrected, as the B_{12} in supplements is in a free form and doesn't require separation.

Options for B_{12} replacement include tablets, sublingual (under the tongue) liquids and injections. I prefer the sublingual route as there may be advantages for those with absorption issues and it is more convenient than injections.

Sublingual doses of 1 mg (1000 mcg) to 3 mg (3000 mcg) of B_{12} daily for ten days, then once per week for four weeks, then monthly have been found effective in restoring B_{12} levels in those with deficiency.

Antioxidants

Antioxidants include vitamin C, vitamin E, beta carotene (vitamin A precursor), and the minerals selenium and manganese.

These substances act as free radical scavengers, protecting our bodies from the damage caused by reactive oxygen species that are created by oxidation reactions and damage our cells. As discussed in the "What is an Autoimmune Condition?" chapter, a lack of antioxidants may result in thyroid damage from hydrogen peroxide every time iodine is processed by the thyroid.

The Recommended Daily Allowance (RDA) for foods was established to guide the public on how much of each nutrient was needed to prevent overt disease. However, these numbers were determined decades ago without the benefit of current research and without an adequate understanding of how nutrition affects our physiology. These guidelines have become our "ideals" in nutrient intake. Unfortunately, our RDA for most antioxidants is too low to see the benefits.

For example, vitamin C becomes an antioxidant at doses above 600 mg, while the RDA is only 60 mg, one tenth of that. While 60 mg will prevent scurvy, it will not prevent free radical damage. Vitamin E is an antioxidant at a dose of 200 mg–400 mg (RDA is 10 mg), and selenium should be taken at a dose of 200 mcg–400 mcg for those with Hashimoto's (RDA is 70 mcg). Vitamins C and E can be found in many food sources, but supplementation may also be helpful.

Vitamin A, however, when taken as a supplement, can be toxic in excessive amounts, and should only be taken from food sources. Carrots, pumpkin, and sweet potatoes are the richest source of beta carotene, the precursor of vitamin A. They won't cause any harm, except for a potential yellowing of the skin, known as carotenosis (seriously!). At this point we will know that we have enough vitamin A as our body will stop converting the beta carotene to the vitamin A. The extra beta carotene is stored in our fat cells until it is ready to be converted to vitamin A. The yellowing of the skin is reversible upon limiting our intake of foods rich in beta carotene. Yellowing of the skin is more common in people with hypothyroidism, who may have an impaired ability to convert the beta carotene due to lack of thyroid hormones. If your skin turns yellow, this is of course a sign to cut back on carrots, pumpkin, and sweet potatoes.

Selenium

In normal thyroid function, iodide from food sources will trigger the production of hydrogen peroxide so that the iodide can be converted to its usable iodine form. The reactive hydrogen peroxide causes oxidative damage that is neutralized by the antioxidant selenium, which is also a necessary building block in thyroid synthesis.

However, in the presence of excess iodide intake, more hydrogen peroxide will be produced, requiring more selenium for neutralization. Coupled with selenium deficiency, one can understand that excessive iodine intake can lead to dangerous levels of hydrogen peroxide production. When the reactive hydrogen peroxide causes oxidative damage and inflammation of the surrounding thyroid tissues, this inflammation triggers lymphocytes or white blood cells (WBCs), to converge and clean up.

As the WBCs are converging, small amounts of antibodies will be formed to help mark the damaged cells that need to be cleaned up. Mouse models have been found to have spontaneously occurring low levels of circulating TPO antibodies, which I theorize serve a clean-up function. According to some professionals, in instances of higher turnover of cells seen with excess oxidative damage due to iodine excess and selenium deficiency, more antibodies are produced and an immune system shift can be induced, resulting in the failure to recognize self from non-self. This is how autoimmunity starts. Thus, selenium deficiency has also been recognized as a risk factor for Hashimoto's.

More iodine→More H_2O_2→Not enough selenium/glutathione to neutralize→Lots of cells with oxidative damage→Inflammation and convergence of WBCs→Excessive amount of antibodies form to mark damaged cells →Immune shift→Self-recognition impaired (autoimmunity)

According to the National Institutes of Health, most cases of selenium deficiency are associated with severe gastrointestinal problems such as Crohn's disease or surgical removal of the stomach, however, selenium deficiency may also occur in celiac disease and other inflammatory bowel disorders due to the malabsorption from damage to the small intestine.

The co-occurrence of Hashimoto's and celiac has been clearly established. I would even venture to say that one does not need to have full-blown celiac to have an impaired absorption of selenium.

Selenium plays a very important role in thyroid function:
1) Acting as catalyst to convert the inactive T4 to the biologically active T3
2) Protecting thyroid cells from oxidative damage from hydrogen peroxide by forming selenoproteins

Three specific diseases have been associated with selenium deficiency:
- Keshan disease is found in selenium-deficient children and is associated with an enlarged and malfunctioning heart.
- Kashin-Beck disease, which causes bone malformation, is found when iodine and selenium are both deficient.
- Myxedematous Endemic Cretinism results in intellectual disability. Scar tissue is seen in place of the thyroid.

Note: Myexedema: mucin and edema. Mucin is a substance that accumulates in hypothyroidism.

Studies have proposed that supplemental selenium could alleviate toxic effect of excessive iodine intake on the thyroid.

Selenium is a trace mineral that is incorporated into proteins to make antioxidants like glutathione peroxidase. This type of protein is known as a selenoprotein, and prevents damage from hydrogen peroxide generated from the conversion of iodide to iodine by breaking down the hydrogen peroxide into water particles. This allows for the removal of the cells affected by oxidative damage, leads to the preservation of tissue integrity and prevents the convergence of white blood cells. [15]

$$H_2O_2 + \textit{Glutathione Peroxidase} \rightarrow H_2O \textit{ (water)}$$

However, in the presence of excessive iodine, a relative selenium deficiency occurs. Since glutathione peroxidase is made of selenium, the enzyme activity will be compromised when selenium is depleted. According to Xu, et. al., "Selenium supplements alleviate damage of TPO that results from iodine excess." The scar tissue seen in the selenium-deficient children affected with myxedematous endemic cretinism further supports the notion that a lack of the antioxidant selenium leads to the destruction of thyroid tissue due to inability to neutralize the hydrogen peroxide.

In a study done with mice that developed autoimmune thyroiditis induced by iodine, this development was prevented when selenium was given. Selenium reduced the TgAb titers and increased the number of circulating T regulatory cells that help the immune system recognize itself and prevent the lymphocytic (WBC) infiltration of the thyroid cells that is present in autoimmune thyroiditis.

A study in Africa showed that two months of selenium supplementation restored the glutathione peroxidase activity, and improved thyroid function through increased conversion of T4 to the active T3.

A similar study found that selenium intake protects against thyroid autoimmunity by acting as an antioxidant, and also has an effect on HLA-DR gene expression, further preventing autoimmunity. Furthermore, ultrasounds of the thyroid following selenium supplementation showed reduced lesions in the thyroid gland.

The RDA for selenium has been defined as 55 mcg in the United States, and an upper limit of 400 mcg has been suggested. A study done in South Dakota did not find any signs of toxicity at levels as high as 724 mcg, however, changes in nail structure, a sign of toxicity, were reported with selenium intake of 900 mcg per day in China. Most reported toxicity cases have been associated with industrial accidents and manufacturing errors. Some symptoms of selenium toxicity that have been reported include GI disturbances, hair loss, changes in hair and nails, peripheral neuropathy, fatigue, irritability, garlic-smelling breath, and a jaundice-like yellow tint to the skin.

While it may be tempting to increase selenium intake by increasing consumption of selenium-rich foods such as Brazil nuts, it is important to realize that selenium content varies widely for foods grown in different soils. While the Dakotas have selenium-rich soils, other areas such as Russia and China have deficient levels of selenium.

Again, importation of foods further complicates these issues. The amounts of selenium in a single Brazil nut have been reported to range tenfold depending on where the nut was grown. This means there could be anywhere from 55 mcg to 550 mcg per ounce of nuts. Additionally, absorption issues due to GI problems may limit the availability of selenium from food sources.

While the RDA of selenium may often be found in multivitamin/mineral combinations, that will not be sufficient for TPOAb reduction. Studies have been done to test the minimal dose of selenium for TPO antibody reduction, and that dose was established to be 200 mcg daily, even a 100 mcg dose did not produce a statistically significant TPO antibody reduction. The bioavailability of minerals is very delicate and can be greatly affected by food or the presence of other substances.

Multivitamin supplements also have so many different ingredients that the absorption of this important mineral may be reduced. I recommend taking the selenium on an empty stomach with vitamin E, which works in synergy with selenium, to ensure proper absorption.

Ferritin

Iron is necessary for transporting oxygen throughout our bodies. It is necessary for cell growth and differentiation. Iron deficiency leads to limited oxygen delivery to cells causing fatigue, difficulty concentrating, and reduced immune function. A deficiency in iron is one potential cause of anemia.

Your doctor may test for anemia by running a panel for red blood cells, hemoglobin, hematocrit, and iron levels, and all of them may come up normal. However, you may still be anemic. If not enough iron is available, the body may pull the iron from less important physiological processes, such as hair growth, to keep enough iron circulating in the blood.

Ferritin is the name given to your body's iron reserve protein. Ferritin is required for transport of T3 to cell nuclei and for the utilization of the T3 hormone.

Ferritin deficiency is the primary cause of hair loss in premenopausal women, and is often the reason behind why women with Hashimoto's continue to lose hair despite normal thyroid levels.

Ferritin hair loss presents as increased hair loss during shampooing and brushing, as well as overall thinning of hair without specific pattern or bald spots. Rather, the woman may find that her hair feels thinner all over, and is less dense.

Ferritin levels can also be measured and will be a better predictor of how much iron you have stored in your body and available for use. Ferritin should be checked in all women with Hashimoto's, and in anyone experiencing hair loss.

In addition to poor intake of dietary iron rich foods and lack of hydrochloric acid, pregnancy (due to increased need for iron) and heavy menstruation increase the risk of iron/ferritin deficiency. During each menstruation, a woman will lose 10–15 mg of iron, while a pregnancy may cause a loss of 600–1000 mg of iron.

As iron needs an acid presence to be absorbed, antacids and calcium supplements taken around mealtimes may reduce the absorption of iron from foods and supplements.

Anyone with hair loss and taking PPI's or acid suppressing medications should immediately get his/her ferritin levels checked.

Dietary factors can also impact iron levels. Tannins in tea and coffee can inhibit iron absorption and should be spaced out by an hour from iron-containing meals. Phytates found in nuts, legumes, and grains may also affect iron absorption, as well as egg whites.

Normal ferritin levels for women are between 12 and 150 ng/mL. Ferritin levels of at least 40 ng/ml are required to stop hair loss, while levels of at least 70 ng/ml are needed for hair regrowth. The optimal ferritin level for thyroid function is between 90-110 ng/ml.

Iron is present in the heme and nonheme version in foods. The heme version is the better absorbed version and is found primarily in animal products. The highest levels of iron are found in organ meats … yes, delicious liver. Beef, turkey, and chicken are the next best choices. (Sorry to all of my vegetarian friends.) In contrast, nonheme iron is found in nuts, beans, and spinach and is not usually absorbed as well.

To restore your iron levels, you can eat cooked liver twice per week or eat beef a few times per week. Vitamin C increases the absorption of iron, so taking a vitamin C tablet or vitamin C rich food such as broccoli along with an iron-rich food is the best way to increase iron and ferritin levels. Creating an acidic environment by taking a Betaine and Pepsin supplement with meals can be helpful as well.

Most iron supplements are in the non-heme form and thus may not be absorbed as well. Additionally, many people find that they get terrible stomachaches from the supplements, and they find them extremely constipating! If choosing to take iron supplements, do so with much caution as they are one of the leading causes of overdose for children and adults. An iron overdose can be deadly, so make sure you keep the iron out of reach of children. Be sure you speak to your physician or pharmacist about a dose appropriate for you.

Zinc

Zinc is an essential element to our well-being. Zinc acts as a catalyst in about 100 different enzyme reactions required by our body, and is involved in DNA synthesis, immune function, protein synthesis, and cell division. It is required for proper sense of taste and smell, detoxification, wound healing, and thyroid function. Zinc is not stored in the body, thus a daily intake of zinc is required to maintain sufficient levels.

One in four individuals in the general population may be zinc deficient, and most people with hypothyroidism are in fact zinc deficient. Zinc deficiency prevents the conversion of T4 into the active T3 version. This results in a slowed metabolism of proteins. Zinc is also needed to form TSH, and may become depleted in those with hypothyroidism who are constantly producing more TSH.

Zinc deficiency has also been associated with increased intestinal permeability and susceptibility to infections as well as reduced detoxification of bacterial toxins.

Oysters have the highest concentration of zinc, but they are not something most people would enjoy eating every day. Beef, liver, pork, lobster, and chicken are the next best sources of zinc, as it is easiest to extract zinc from meat compared with non-meat sources. Thus, vegetarians also have an increased risk of zinc deficiency.

Absorption of zinc may be impaired by damage from intestinal disease such as celiac disease and other malabsorption syndromes. Phytates found in grains, legumes, nuts and seeds can bind zinc and prevent its absorption when eaten alongside zinc containing foods. Taking iron supplements in conjunction with meals may also prevent the absorption of zinc from food.

Zinc deficiency can show up on a liver function blood test as low alkaline phosphatase levels. Alkaline phosphatase will be discussed in further detail in its very own chapter.

In order to address deficiency, zinc supplementation may be utilized, with doses of no more than 30 mg per day. Zinc supplementation above 40 mg may cause a depletion in copper levels, and thus if choosing to take zinc, one should also take a copper supplement. Usually 1.5 mg–3 mg of copper should be sufficient. (General recommendations are to take 1 mg of copper for every 15 mg of zinc). Caution: Zinc can cause depletion in copper and iron. Fifty milligrams of zinc given over ten weeks impaired both iron and copper absorption in one study.

Symptoms of copper deficiency are: anemia not responsive to iron supplementation, trouble with walking and balance, fatigue, and light headedness.

Amino Acid Deficiency

Proteins are broken down into amino acids, and amino acids are described as the building blocks for our cells. People with Hashimoto's may also be deficient in amino acids because of impaired protein digestion. Free form amino acid supplements may be helpful, however, supplementing with mega doses of amino acids may not always be appropriate.

Tyrosine

Tyrosine is required for production of thyroid hormone and is often used in "Natural Thyroid Supplements" along with iodine. The use of Tyrosine is controversial in Hashimoto's. Tyrosine will increase the production of thyroid hormones, which may be stressful on the adrenals if the adrenals are not supported properly. Small amounts of tyrosine from food sources, elemental formulas or as part of an adrenal supplement might not cause problems, but I would be cautious of high-dose tyrosine supplements.

Glutamine

The amino acid glutamine is usually depleted in people with Hashimoto's and chronic stress. This amino acid is essential to proper gut lining and immune function. (More in the "Gut" chapter).

Testing for Depletions

Standard blood tests may not always reveal vitamin and mineral deficiencies until we are very depleted, as the body will provide these nutrients to the blood as long as it can, pulling them away from less vital parts of our bodies, such as hair. Hair tests may be more sensitive to changes in nutrient levels, and may be ordered by patients themselves. Additionally, some labs specialize in micronutrient testing and can be ordered by physicians. (More information can be found in the "Testing" chapter.)

ANTI-NUTRIENTS

We discussed some examples of foods that contain anti-nutrients that bind vitamins and minerals and prevent them from becoming absorbed in our bodies, such as those found in phytates. These foods can have an impact on thyroid function through depletions of necessary nutrients needed for optimal function.

Other foods can cause poor conversion to active thyroid hormone even in people without autoimmune conditions and in people who have TSH levels in the normal reference range.

Goitrogens

Goitrogens are substances that suppress the thyroid gland by interfering with thyroid hormone production. As a compensatory mechanism, the thyroid will enlarge to counteract the reduced hormone production. This enlargement is also known as a goiter.

You may have heard that you should avoid goitrogenic foods if you have a thyroid condition. This is only partially true, as all goitrogens are not created equally. Different goitrogenic substances are contained in various foods.

Table 5: Goitrogenic Foods

Bamboo shoots
Bok Choy
Brassica genus veggies
Broccoli
Broccolini
Brussels sprouts
Cabbage
Canola Oil
Cassava
Cauliflower
Choy sum
Collard greens
Horseradish
Kale
Kohlrabi
Millet
Mizuna
Mustard greens
Peaches
Peanuts
Pears
Pine nuts
Radishes
Rapeseed
Rapini
Rutabagas
Soy
Spinach
Strawberries
Sweet potato
Tatsoi
Turnips

Cruciferous Vegetables

Cruciferous vegetables such as cabbage, broccoli, and cauliflower contain glucosinolates, substances that block iodine uptake into the thyroid. Eating too many in the raw state can cause symptoms of hypothyroidism in someone with otherwise well controlled symptoms.

Luckily, cruciferous vegetables are only goitrogenic in the raw state. Cooking or lightly steaming will deactivate the glucosinolates, as will fermenting the vegetables (as in sauerkraut), thus diminishing the goitrogenic activity. While consuming fermented and cooked cruciferous vegetables is preferred, occasionally eating small amounts of these foods in the raw states should not aggravate autoimmune thyroid conditions. Canola oil, a goitrogen found in processed foods, should be avoided.

Soy

Soy is one particular goitrogen that is especially detrimental for Hashimoto's patients. The isoflavones genistein, daidzein and glycitein in soy reduce thyroid output by blocking activity of the TPO enzyme.

Soy has been linked with the development of autoimmune thyroid conditions, and children fed soy formula were almost three times more likely to develop anti-thyroid antibodies compared with breast-fed children.

Studies of soy isoflavones in animals suggest possible adverse effects like augmentation of reproductive organs, modulation of endocrine function, and antithyroid effects. Antithyroid effects may also be propagated by increasing the loss of circulating T4 from the blood via bile.

Table 6: Goitrogen Effects On Thyroid

Natural Substances	Agents	Action
Millet, soy	Flavonoids	Impairs thyroperoxidase activity
Cassava, sweet potato, sorghum	Cyanogenic glucosides metabolized to thiocyanates	Inhibits iodine thyroidal uptake
Babassu coconut, mandioca	Flavonoids	Inhibits thyroperoxidase
Cruciferous vegetables: cabbage, cauliflower, broccoli, turnips, canola	Glucosinolates	Impairs iodine thyroidal uptake
Seaweed (kelp)	Iodine excess	Inhibits release of thyroidal hormones
Malnutrition	Vitamin A deficiency	Increases TSH stimulation
	Iron deficiency	Reduces heme-dependent thyroperoxidase thyroidal activity
Selenium	Selenium deficiency	Accumulates peroxides and causes deiodinase deficiency; impairs thyroid hormone synthesis

The goitrogens in soy are still present after cooking; additionally soy is a very common allergen. Thus, people with underactive thyroid function and Hashimoto's should avoid soy completely. On a personal note, I have suffered from a "thyroid crash", feeling drained and exhausted the day after eating soy.

Millet is a cereal crop that is not related to wheat, and it is often used in gluten-free bread and bakery products. However, millet also contains isoflavones that inhibit thyroid peroxidase and should be avoided by people with thyroid disorders.

My personal experience

After learning that selenium helped reduce anti-thyroid antibodies when I was first diagnosed with Hashimoto's, I decided to eat two Brazil nuts per day. While the nuts were yummy, unfortunately, I did not see a change in TPOAb on my next lab test.

However, after starting selenium at 200 mcg, as well as reducing soy intake in the summer of 2011, I soon noticed that I felt so much more calm (a signal of diminished thyrotoxicity).

This feeling was supported by my lab values, which showed a reduction in TPOAb from the mid-800s to the mid-300s.

Chapter Summary

- ✓ Digestion is impaired in Hashimoto's, resulting in depletion of nutrients.
- ✓ Diet, medications, and lifestyle contribute to poor digestion.
- ✓ Check levels of vitamin B_{12}, zinc, ferritin.
- ✓ Replace with supplementation as indicated.

✓ Consider selenium methionine 200 mcg–400 mcg daily.

✓ Consider taking Betaine with Pepsin with protein meals.

✓ Goitrogens are substances found in foods that interfere with thyroid function.

✓ Most goitrogens are inactivated by cooking and fermenting, and can be eaten in moderation.

✓ Goitrogens in soy are still present after cooking and soy should be avoided.

"Poison is in everything, and no thing is without poison. The dosage makes it either a poison or a remedy."~Paracelsus (1493-1541)

7: IODINE CONTROVERSY

The thyroid is very sensitive to iodine levels and has been shown to adapt its physiology based on the available levels of iodine. The relationship between iodine intake and occurrence of thyroid disease has been described to have a U-shape distribution; another Goldilocks supplement!

Researchers in Denmark found that the effect of iodine on hypothyroidism seemed to be U-shaped as well, with rates that were either too low or too high, causing hypothyroidism (too low-goiter, too high-autoimmune). A maximum daily threshold of 150 mcg is recommended.

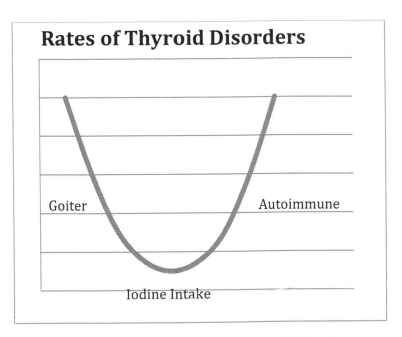

Figure 4: Impact of Iodine on Thyroid Disorders

It is widely known that in cases of severe iodine deficiency, hypothyroidism, goiter, and brain damage will develop. Conversely, several studies have shown that excessive iodine intake can lead to Hashimoto's hypothyroidism, and excess iodine intake is now recognized as an environmental trigger for Hashimoto's.

Hashimoto's was not recognized in the U.S. before the start of the nationwide salt iodization program in 1924. In many other countries, studies have shown that rates of autoimmune thyroiditis increase drastically after salt iodization.

Changes have been observed with the incidence of thyroid disorders with very slight variations in iodine intake. In most cases of mild to moderate iodine deficiency, the thyroid compensates and limits its use of iodine for thyroid hormone production, and still keeps thyroid hormone production normal. In order to achieve this, however, the thyroid gland enlarges (this enlargement is called a goiter).

A pattern of TSH levels dropping with advanced age is observed due to the chronic enlargement and increased thyroid hormone production. Thus, elderly persons in mild-moderate iodine deficient conditions are more likely to develop hyperthyroidism.

In contrast, populations with high iodine intake have been observed to have an increasing TSH and increased rates of hypothyroidism as they age. It is hypothesized that this may also be compensation of the thyroid gland in order to adapt for high iodine levels. Caucasian populations seem to be especially susceptible.

As iodine levels increase, more cell death is seen in the thyroid. Hydrogen peroxide, a reactive oxygen species, is produced in the conversion of iodine to its usable state in the thyroid. The overabundance of hydrogen peroxide leads to damage to thyroid cells. White blood cells (lymphocytes) come to "clean up" these dead thyroid cells.

As thyroid peroxidase (TPO) is the enzyme involved in triggering hydrogen peroxide release, perhaps the TPO enzyme becomes recognized as an "invader," as it keeps causing damage to the surrounding tissues through the release of hydrogen peroxide. The more iodine consumed, the more that needs to be converted, thus signaling more hydrogen peroxide and signaling more lymphocytes to accumulate in the thyroid.

Perhaps there is a threshold of thyroid tissue damage as a result of hydrogen peroxide released that causes our body to recognize this physiological process as a foreign invader.

Excess Iodine Problematic

Excess iodine causes the thyroid to temporarily decrease function to protect against hyperthyroidism (Wolff-Chaikoff effect), which is a protective mechanism. Hypothyroidism attributed to the Wolff-Chaikoff effect does not have an autoimmune component.

Various studies have cited both autoimmune thyroiditis as well as non-autoimmune hypothyroidism resulting from iodine excess.

Researchers in Iran were able to document the rates of thyroid peroxidase antibodies (TPOAb) and thyroglobulin antibodies (TgAb) before and after a national salt iodization program started in 1994. In 1983-84, positive TPOAb and positive TgAb were found in 3.2% and 4% of the 465 adults selected for random sampling in Tehran.

This sampling was repeated with 1,426 adults in Tehran again in 1999-2000, this time 12.5% were positive for TPOAb and 16.8% were positive for TgAb. The addition of iodine essentially quadrupled the rates of Hashimoto's over a five to six-year span!

Studies in Greece, China, Sri Lanka, and Italy reported similar increases in Hashimoto's after addition of iodine to salt.

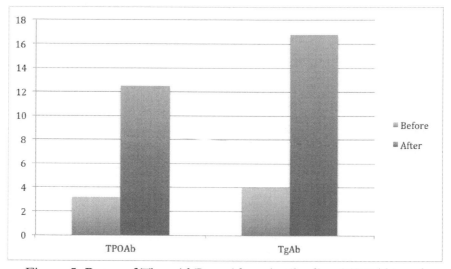

Figure 5: Rates of Thyroid Peroxidase Antibodies (TPOAb) and Thyroglobulin Antibodies (TgAb) in Tehran, Iran before and after a national salt iodization program

The more iodine, the higher the rates of Hashimoto's.

Iodine seems to have a dose responsive effect. A Slovenian study followed the rates of thyroid disorders after the amount of potassium iodide added to the Slovenian salt supply was increased from 10 mg/kg of salt to 25 mg/kg in 1999. This increase resulted in a significant change in the incidence of thyroid disorders. While there was a marked decline in the incidence of iodine deficiency hypothyroidism (goiter), the rates of Hashimoto's more than doubled from the baseline after the increase.

Even Small Amounts of Iodine Can Worsen Hashimoto's

In Germany, a low dose of potassium iodide (250 mcg), was given to forty people who tested positive for anti-thyroid (TPO) antibodies and/or had a thyroid ultrasound showing a hypoechogenic pattern that is consistent with Hashimoto's. A group of forty-three subjects with similar characteristics served as a control group.

Nine patients from the iodine group developed thyroid abnormalities, compared with only one person from the control group. Of the nine patients in the iodine arm, seven developed subclinical hypothyroidism, one became hypothyroid and another hyperthyroid.

Changes were also seen in levels of TPO antibodies as well as on ultrasound of the thyroid. Three of the seven subclinical hypothyroid patients and the hyperthyroid patient regained normal thyroid function after iodine withdrawal.

Considering that iodine increases the rates of Hashimoto's incidence, and even small doses of iodine can lead to the progression of thyroid abnormalities over a short period of time, it is no surprise that 1 in 5 women will have a thyroid dysfunction at some time in her life in the presence of iodized salt.

Also not surprising is the fact that today, 90%-99% of hypothyroidism cases in the United States are due to Hashimoto's, while hypothyroidism due to iodine deficiency is rarely reported.

But I Thought Iodine was Necessary for Hormone Production?

It is. Approximately 52 mcg of iodine needs to be taken up daily by the thyroid gland to produce thyroid hormones.

The U.S. RDA for iodine is 150 mcg for adults who are not pregnant,

220 mcg for pregnant women, 290 mcg for lactating women and 90–120 mcg/day for children from ages 1–13. An upper limit of iodine intake has been set for 1,100 mcg. However, study participants who took 400 mcg of iodine a day began developing subclinical hypothyroidism.

Most guidelines now state that the doses at which adverse events to iodine will occur may vary, and that people with autoimmune thyroid disease may experience adverse effects with iodine intakes considered safe for the general population.

Thus, iodine intake seems to have a very narrow therapeutic index. Some studies have even shown that having a slight deficiency is protective from developing Hashimoto's.

How Much Iodine am I Getting?

While the average American may consume between 6 and 10 grams of salt per day, largely due to processed foods, it is difficult to estimate the amount of iodine that is contained in the Standard American Diet, due to uncertainty of whether the prepared food was made with iodized salt or non-iodized salt.

The FDA estimated that between 2003 and 2004, the average iodine intake in the United States ranged from 138 mcg to 353 mcg per day. However, this data did not consider added iodine that people obtain from the use of iodized salt.

Proponents of high-dose iodine diets and regimens will often cite that Japan, a country with the highest iodine intake, averages 1,000-3,000 µg/day, but has a lower incidence of chronic diseases. However, incidence rates of Hashimoto's in Japan and the U.S. are reported to be similar.[29] Interestingly, an association with one particular gene was found to contribute to the development of

Hashimoto's in Japanese, but not in American, subjects. So perhaps, Japanese are genetically better adapted to high iodine intake compared with Caucasian populations.

Test to Measure Iodine Status

More than 90% of dietary iodine is excreted in urine, thus dietary iodine intake can be measured through a urinary iodine test. Spot urine iodine measurements are a useful and relatively easy tool to measure iodine status. ZRT labs (more information in the "Testing" chapter) allows people in most states to order their own spot urinary iodine tests.

Sources of Iodine

In addition to iodized salt, which is estimated to contain 47.5 mcg of iodine per gram of salt (or 285 mcg of iodine per teaspoon), other sources of iodine include seaweed (kelp, nori, kombu, wakame), seafood, dairy products (due to the use of iodine sanitizing agents in the dairy industry as well as iodine containing feed), grains, and eggs (due to the iodine content of the feed of the hens).

Plants may also contain iodine and the amount will vary based on the iodine content in the soil or use of iodine-containing fertilizers. Areas close to the oceans generally have more iodine rich soils compared to the inland and mountainous regions.

Importation of foods can make estimates challenging. One source of iodine that is often missed is spirulina, the blue-green algae touted for its health benefits. For a full listing of estimated iodine content of various foods, please refer to the assessment at the end of this chapter.

Table 7: Sample of Food Sources of Iodine

Food	Approximate Micrograms (mcg) per serving	Percent DV*
Seaweed, whole or sheet, 1 g	16 to 2,984	11% to 1,989%
Cod, baked, 3 ounces	99	66%
Yogurt, plain, low-fat, 1 cup	75	50%
Iodized salt, 1.5 g (approx. 1/4 teaspoon)	71	47%
Milk, reduced fat, 1 cup	56	37%
Fish sticks, 3 ounces	54	36%
Bread, white, enriched, 2 slices	45	30%
Fruit cocktail in heavy syrup, canned, 1/2 cup	42	28%
Shrimp, 3 ounces	35	23%
Ice cream, chocolate, 1/2 cup	30	20%
Macaroni, enriched, boiled, 1 cup	27	18%
Egg, 1 large	24	16%
Tuna, canned in oil, drained, 3 ounces	17	11%
Corn, cream style, canned, 1/2 cup	14	9%
Prunes, dried, 5 prunes	13	9%
Cheese, cheddar, 1 ounce	12	8%
Raisin Bran cereal, 1 cup	11	7%
Lima beans, mature, boiled, 1/2 cup	8	5%
Apple juice, 1 cup	7	5%
Green peas, frozen, boiled, 1/2 cup	3	2%
Banana, 1 medium	3	2%

Table from: http://ods.od.nih.gov/factsheets/Iodine-HealthProfessional/

In addition to dietary sources, iodine can also be found in medications like amiodarone (a recognized trigger for Hashimoto's) and in over-the-counter multivitamin supplements, prenatal vitamins, and of course, iodine supplements.

Formulations that promise to "boost thyroid function," "aid a sluggish thyroid," etc., often contain high doses of iodine and should not be used by those with acute autoimmune hypothyroidism.

Processed foods, such as cured meats, cakes, pies, instant mixes, garlic salts, artificial dyes, (especially Red Dye No. 3), also contain iodine and should be avoided by those who wish to adhere to a low-iodine diet.

Iodine in the Standard American Diet

Let's do the math, starting with a breakfast that is considered "healthy" by our SAD (Standard American Diet) standards. (Note: pun definitely intended!)

Breakfast	Iodine
1 cup milk	56 mcg
Raisin Bran Cereal	11 mcg
Banana	3 mcg

Lunch	
Yogurt	75 mcg
Bread (2 pieces):	90 mcg
Cheddar cheese	12 mcg
Canned Tuna	17 mcg

That's 264 mcg of iodine before dinner...

What if you took your multivitamin?

A Centrum® multivitamin contains 150 mcg of iodine.

Now you are up to 414mcg...

What about those of us who like to add salt to our food?

You can add 71 mcg for every ¼ teaspoon ... 485mcg.

What about going out for sushi?

Combining the seaweed and the fish can easily bring your intake to 1000 mcg, if not more

What if you wanted ice cream for dessert?

You get the picture. The Standard American Diet exceeds the threshold of safe iodine consumption for those with autoimmune thyroid conditions.

Controversy

Whether Hashimoto's patients should avoid iodine, take iodine, or ignore iodine, has been a controversial topic in the autoimmune thyroid community. Proponents of using high doses of iodine claim that studies done in animals showed that inorganic iodines did not induce autoimmune thyroiditis unless they were combined with goitrogens. However, a review of the literature will produce many other studies that have shown the opposite to be true. [3]

In experimental mouse models of autoimmune thyroiditis, mice spontaneously developed low levels of antibodies to TPO, which I interpret to be a normal physiological "clean-up" state. When iodine is added to the water of mice, the prevalence and severity of autoimmune thyroiditis increase markedly. In fact, excess iodine is used to stimulate autoimmune thyroiditis in animal models.

Additionally, one study done in Korea showed that iodine restriction alone can recover hypothyroid Hashimoto's patients to a euthyroid state within three months! This study was done on ninety patients who were randomized to either continue ingesting the same amount of iodine or restrict their iodine intake to less than 100 mcg per day. 78% of people in the iodine restriction group regained normal thyroid function manifested by a normal TSH value within three months.

Predicative factors of recovery were lower initial TSH as well as higher initial iodine excretion.

Factors predicative of recovery of thyroid function after three months of iodine restriction
Shorter disease duration TSH level closer to normal reference range Higher iodine levels at baseline

The authors report that the patients in the study group who did not recover normal TSH at the conclusion of the three-month trial did show a decreasing trend in TSH, and predicted that they too would become euthyroid if given more time.

Interestingly, 45.5% of the control group recovered normal function as well. This is a much higher rate than the 20% of people who reportedly revert to normal thyroid function with Hashimoto's. The authors were not sure if some members of the control group decided to restrict iodine intake on their own or if other variables accounted for this high number. The authors recommended that iodine restriction should be a first-line measure for those with Hashimoto's hypothyroidism, before thyroid supplemental medication is started.

While I think this sounds like a compelling reason to throw away your box of iodized salt, a few things should be noted about this study.

1) The TPO value was only measured at baseline, and not at the three-month follow-up.
2) Echogenic studies were not done to compare the baseline/three-month follow-up lesions in the thyroid.
3) Sources of iodine were not examined to rule out possible cross-contaminating effects of halogens such as fluorine and bromine, which may be found in kelp, seaweed and other iodine-rich foods traditionally eaten in Korea.
4) Selenium levels were not assessed during the study.

Interaction of Halogens with Iodine

Our threshold for iodine consumption can be affected by halogens such as chlorine, bromine, and fluorine. The binding structures or the "business end" of these molecules may look very similar to the binding structure of iodine.

Storage proteins, enzymes, and transporters in our bodies that bind to our micronutrients have a predefined limited capacity. An excess of other molecules with similar chemical structures may occupy all of the sites that are usually reserved for processing iodine. This is the basis of modern pharmacology, and how most drug-to-drug interactions occur. When halogens occupy the designated iodine binding sites, a change in absorption, distribution, metabolism, or excretion of iodine may occur which can lead to toxicity, even at "normal" therapeutic amounts. (More information about halogens will be covered in the "Toxins" chapter.)

ASSESSMENT: How much iodine are you getting from foods?

(Adapted from http://foodhealth.info/iodine/)

Foods Highest in Iodine	Iodine (mcg)
Seaweed, whole or sheet	160–29,840
Salt, iodized	1,855
Cod liver, canned	500
Oil, cod liver	400
Sardine filets in olive oil, canned, drained	400
Broth or bouillon, beef, dehydrated	390
Cod, Atlantic, raw	360
Pâté, fish or shellfish	310
Haddock, steamed	260
Fish mousse	250
Haddock, breaded, fried	250
Haddock, smoked	250
Herring, smoked, in oil	200
Soup, seafood	198
Mullet, baked	190
Squid, fried	173
Cod, baked	130
Cod, salted, poached	130
Lobster, boiled	130
Mackerel, fried	130
Crustacean or mollusk (average)	123
Fish nugget, fried	120
Caviar	117
Whelk, cooked	114
Cod, steamed	110
Fish cake, frozen, raw	110
Mussel, boiled	106
Oyster, Pacific, raw	101
Crab, cooked	100
Mackerel, baked	100

*Iodine content is per 100 grams of food weight

Foods with High Amounts of Iodine	Iodine (mcg)
Mackerel, smoked	98
Egg yolk, cooked	89
Milk, skim, powder	85
Sardine, in oil, canned, drained	80
Clam, cooked	80
Ling, raw	80
Milk, semi-skim, powder	80
Periwinkle	80
Milk, whole, powder	71
Whiting, steamed	70
Kebab, fish	68
Custard, English cream	67
Herring, grilled	67
Sardine, in tomato sauce, canned, drained	67
Smelt, raw	67
Chocolate mousse	66
Milk, semi-skim, flavored	66
Semolina pudding	65
Spiny lobster, cooked	65
Pilchard, in tomato sauce, canned	64
Fish, cooked (average)	62
Caviar substitute, Lumpfish eggs	60
Crab, canned	60
Fish in sauce, frozen	60
Gnocchi, potato	60
Milk, skim, vitamin fortified	60
Sea bass, raw	60
Soy yogurt, flavored	60
Tiramisu	60
Whiting, fried	60
Cereal bar, low-calorie	53

*Iodine content is per 100 grams of food weight.

Foods with Moderate Amounts of Iodine	Iodine (mcg)
Egg, poached	52
Egg, scrambled	52
Omelet, plain	52
Apple crumble	50
Cheese, Roquefort	50
Dark chocolate, 70% cocoa	50
Fruit charlotte, from bakery	50
Salmon in puff pastry	50
Sauce, hollandaise	50
Sauce, pesto	50
Blue cheese, de Bresse	48
Cheese, Rouy	48
Sandwich on French bread, smoked salmon, butter	46
Anglerfish or monkfish, grilled	45
Crayfish, raw	45
Egg, fried, salted	45
Tuna, cooked	45
Omelet with herbs	45
Omelet, cheese	44
Salmon, farmed, raw	44
Scallop, Great Atlantic, with coral, raw	43
Cheese, Edam	42
Vol-au-vent with seafood	42
Scampi, fried	41
Herring, smoked	40
Omelet with bacon	40
Salmon, smoked	40
Soy yogurt with fruit	40
Trout, smoked	40
Tuna, raw	40
Mackerel, in tomato sauce, canned	40

*Iodine content is per 100 grams of food weight.

Foods Rich in Iodine	Iodine (mcg)
Egg, hard boiled	39
Egg, soft boiled	39
Egg, whole, raw	39
Cheese, goat, Crottin	39
Herring, fried	38
Salmon, carpaccio	38
Beaufort cheese	38
Omelet with mushrooms	37
Cheese, Cheddar	37
Cheese, Livarot	37
Shrimp or prawn, cooked	37
Ice cream in cone	36
Cheese, Pont l'Eveque	35
Chocolate powder, sweetened, enriched	35
Eggnog	35
Soup, cream of tomato	35

*Iodine content is per 100 grams of food weight

Chapter Summary

✓ Iodine perpetuates the autoimmune attack.
✓ Check iodine levels
✓ If normal/high iodine levels, consider limiting iodine to <100 mcg per day for three months and then retesting TPO antibodies

My Personal Experience With Iodine

Since I have been my own human guinea pig, I tested iodine supplements on myself, and unfortunately noticed an increase in thyrotoxic symptoms following high iodine intake (thyrotoxicity results from thyroid tissue destruction).

Others have reported an increase in TPO antibodies following eating more iodine-rich foods. I personally had my iodine levels tested and was in the mid-normal range at the time.

Based on my experiment, I have concluded that while I fully agree with proponents of high-dose iodine that iodine is important for breast health and breast cancer prevention, I disagree with the assertion that all thyroid patients are deficient in iodine and need to be on high-dose supplements.

In a recent interview Dr. David Brownstein, a proponent of high-dose iodine and author of the excellent book "Overcoming Thyroid Disorders", stated that iodine can aggravate autoimmune thyroid conditions and that iodine can be "akin to pouring gas over a fire."

I suspect that high-dose iodine does not actually *cause* Hashimoto's, but is simply too much to handle for an overburdened system, and thus iodine perpetuates the vicious cycle of thyroid destruction.

Perhaps once the other leaks are fixed (deficiencies, adrenals, gut), the iodine will no longer proliferate Hashimoto's. More about this in the upcoming chapters!

"Something, somewhere is causing inflammation in your body, which leads to an immune imbalance."

8: INFLAMMATION

Inflammation is present in most autoimmune conditions and can trigger adrenal fatigue as well as an autoimmune cascade. There may be a multitude of reasons for inflammation in the body, including infections, food intolerances, injuries, intestinal flora, and a pro-inflammatory environment created by an imbalanced omega-3 and omega-6 ratio. Thus, in order to restore balance we need to be sure that we are promoting an anti-inflammatory environment.

Our bodies require the essential omega-3 and omega-6 fats, and their ratio should be 1:1 for proper immune function. Omega-3 fatty acids reduce inflammation, while omega-6 fatty acids promote inflammation. While inflammation serves a protective purpose to our bodies, in excess, it can be problematic. Most Americans get too many omega-6 essential fatty acids and not enough omega-3 essential fatty acids.

Omega-6 acids are most often found in our diet through the consumption of vegetable oils, nuts and seeds. Vegetable oils include canola, corn, soybean, peanut, sunflower, safflower, cottonseed, grapeseed, margarine, and shortening.

These same oils are often found in processed foods such as salad dressing, store-bought condiments, mayonnaise, chips, artificial cheese, store-bought roasted nuts, cookies, crackers, snack foods, sauces, and almost everything in the middle aisles of the grocery store.

Vegetable oils and margarine were recommended for years as a healthful and cheap alternative to saturated fats, however, they have now been recognized to be dangerous to human health and should be eliminated from the diet.

Vegetable oils have a very high level of omega-6 acids, and eating them can cause an imbalance. Omega-6 acids can easily oxidize not only in body cells, but also when exposed to heat or light. These oxidized fats can cause inflammation and mutation in cells and also increase the risk of cancer.

Meanwhile, saturated fats like butter, lard, and animal fats have been getting a bad rap. However, these traditional foods are likely a better choice than the inflammatory vegetable oils.

A study conducted at the University of Western Ontario has shown that people who eat more saturated fats in their diets have a lower risk of cancer than those with the least amount of saturated fats in the diet! (Bring on the lard!)

Another study concluded that eating polyunsaturated fats (like those in vegetable oils) could stimulate cancer, while saturated fat protects against cancer and reduces inflammation.

Vegetable oils and margarine were only introduced into our diets in the last century. Traditional natural oil preparation methods like pressing or separating (think olive oil) does not extract vegetable oils from vegetables like corn and soybeans. Vegetable oils are manufactured in a factory and the oil is chemically removed from crops and then altered. For example, canola oil is made from rapeseed, and a petroleum solvent is used to extract this oil. Many vegetable oils are also often made from genetically modified crops and they contain large amounts of pesticides.

When diets high in polyunsaturated fats were tested on animals, it was concluded that they can cause problems with learning, are toxic to the liver, are responsible for malfunction of the immune system, slow mental and physical growth, cause chromosomal damage, and premature aging. In addition, diets high in polyunsaturated fat are responsible for increased rates of cancer, heart disease, and weight gain.

Omega 3

Promoting a better omega-3 to omega-6 ratio through eating more foods rich in omega-3 fatty acids in addition to reducing the intake of omega-6 fatty acids may be helpful in restoring immune balance.

Omega-3 acids are found primarily in fish, shellfish and flaxseeds, and can also be taken in supplement form for those who cannot eat adequate amounts of fish or are concerned about mercury content.

Omega-3 acid supplementation has been found to be helpful in a variety of autoimmune conditions. Doses of 1–4 grams are recommended when taking fish oil supplements.

The omega acid content of various meats depends on the type of diet the animals received. Grass-fed organic beef has fewer omega-6s compared with soybean- or corn-fed cattle.

Healthful Oils

The three oils that are recommended for people with Hashimoto's are coconut oil, extra-virgin olive oil, and cod liver oil.

Coconut oil is a saturated fat made up of medium chain fatty acids that may be beneficial to people with underactive thyroids. It can increase metabolism and promote weight loss when substituted for unsaturated fats, and also functions as an antioxidant.

Which Foods are High in Omega-6 Fatty Acids?

Foods with High Percent of Calories from Omega-6 Fatty Acids

>50% (Highest)	20-50% (Higher)	10-20% (High)
Grapeseed oil	Sesame oil	Chicken Fat
Corn oil	Pepitas	Almond
Walnuts	Margarine	Canola Oil
Cottonseed oil	Pecans	Flaxseed Oil
Soybean oil	Peanut Butter	Cashews
	Pistachios	Duck Fat
		Bacon grease
		Lard

Foods With Low to Moderate Amounts of Omega-6 Fatty Acids
(percentages of total calories that come from omega-6)

Lowest (<2%)	Low (2-5%)	Moderate (5-10%)
Coconut oil	Corn	Olive oil
Ribs	Sunflower oil	Goose fat
Milk	Butter	Avocado
Beef	Beef	Olives
Macadamia nuts	Cream	Bacon
Chicken (no skin)	Cocoa butter	Eggs
Lamb	Carrots	Pork chops
Cheese	Macadamia nuts	Popcorn
Grits	Brown rice	Oats
Beets	Flour	
Coconut milk		
Rice		
Salmon		
Yams		
Potatoes		
Seafood		

It may be beneficial for people with hypothyroidism to include coconut oil in their daily diet to increase energy and promote a healthy weight. Four tablespoons daily seems to be the optimal amount for adults. Coconut oil can replace butter in many delicious recipes and can be added to tea in place of cream. It also has a moisturizing effect on the skin when taken internally. Supermodel Miranda Kerr credits her gorgeous skin and hair to consuming 4 tablespoons of coconut oil daily!

Coconut oil is very stable, because of medium chain triglycerides, and it does not produce trans fats when heated, so it is the oil of choice for cooking and frying. Additionally, coconut oil has antiviral, antifungal, and antibacterial properties.

Extra-virgin olive oil is high in monounsaturated fat and low in polyunsaturated fats and is recommended for salad dressing and mayonnaise. It should not be used for cooking or frying, because monounsaturated fat can oxidize in high temperatures.

Cod liver oil is a great source of omega-3 fatty acids and can be used as a dressing, rather than for cooking.

Lab Tests For Inflammation

C-reactive protein and homocysteine are non-specific markers of inflammation and can be ordered as blood tests.

Chapter Summary

✓ Processed vegetable oils promote inflammation.
✓ Use coconut oil, extra-virgin olive oil, and cod liver oil.
✓ Consider taking a fish oil supplement.

"Sickness comes on horseback but departs on foot." ~Dutch Proverb

9: INFECTIONS

When working to identify the root cause, we keep asking questions until we find the answer. So we now know that hypothyroidism occurs because of thyroid destruction, and that thyroid destruction occurs because of self-antibodies. So why does the immune system make self-antibodies?

Let's explore the current autoimmune theories.

Classical autoimmune theories have purported the role of pathogens in the development of autoimmune conditions.

Molecular mimicry

In addition to oxidative damage caused by iodine excess, immune cells may also be attracted to the thyroid as a result of a viral/bacterial infection that either infects the thyroid cells and needs to be cleared, or looks similar to the thyroid cells, causing "molecular mimicry."

An antigen is a substance that evokes the production of antibodies.

Molecular mimicry is the theory that bacterial cells or other microbial "triggers" have a similar appearance to the cells that make up parts of our physiology or "self" antigens.

When an infection occurs, these infectious cells are recognized as foreign. This is really great for getting rid of the infections, but sometimes the immune system targets proteins in the infectious cells that resemble the proteins in our own cells. This inadvertently causes a cross-reaction with our "self" antigens, i.e., our own cells. This case of mistaken identity is thought to trigger the start of autoimmunity.

One example is Streptococcus pyogenes. This is the bacteria that causes the common throat infection known as "strep throat". In some cases, especially when the infection is not treated with antibiotics within two to three weeks, the immune system will start launching an attack against the Streptococcus bacteria.

Unfortunately, a component of the bacteria's cell wall resembles that of the human heart valves, and this results in the immune system attacking the human heart valves in a case of mistaken identity. This reaction is known as rheumatic fever and can be deadly and often necessitates heart valve transplants. Arnold Schwarzenegger is probably the most well-known person who was affected with this condition and has had to have heart valve transplants as a result.

Bystander Effect

The "Bystander Effect" is another classical autoimmune theory that suggests bacteria expose our "self" antigens to the immune system by damaging them during an infection. In this case, the "self" becomes guilty by association and a target for the immune system.

This theory suggests that the autoimmunity may have resulted from an infection of the thyroid by a virus that caused damage of thyroid cells. In many cases, the infections may be "silent," without the person knowing they actually have an infection. This first infection kicks off the autoimmune process.

It is possible that these types of infections start off as transient thyroid inflammation, such as in silent thyroiditis, but under the right conditions turn into chronic cases of autoimmune thyroiditis like Hashimoto's. We will explore these reasons in subsequent chapters.

Infections

Various pathogens have been suggested to play a role in the development of Hashimoto's, ranging from bacteria to viruses to fungi and parasites. Dr. Trevor Marshall, PhD, suggests that it is not merely one type of bacteria or virus that triggers the autoimmune process, but a combination of pathogens present, sometimes compounded by a missing commensal species that determines the type of autoimmune disease that develops.

Bug A + Bug B = Disease C

Bug D + Bug E - Bug F = Disease G

Dr. Marshall and colleagues have found various viral, bacterial, and fungal antigens present in saliva of people with autoimmune conditions. These people do not show signs/symptoms of being infected, yet the agent is taking cover in their bodies.

Which bacteria and viruses have been associated with triggering Hashimoto's?

A variety of bacterial infections have been implicated in triggering autoimmune thyroiditis, including Helicobacter Pylori (the same bacteria that causes ulcers), Borrelia burgdorferi (associated with Lyme disease) and Yersinia enterocolitica.

Antibodies to Yersinia (indicating exposure) in people with Hashimoto's were found fourteen times more often than in people without Hashimoto's. Yersinia membranes contain a site that binds TSH, making it a prime suspect based on the molecular mimicry theory. Infection with this bacteria can induce antibodies against sites that recognize and stimulate TSH receptors, like the TPO or thyroglobulin. People can contract a Yersinia enterocolitica infection from contaminated meat, poultry, dairy products, and seafood (especially oysters). In 2012, a consumer group found that 67% of pork sold in the U.S. was contaminated with Yersinia.

Physicians can run blood tests or breath tests for H. Pylori. Borrelia is available as a blood test, while presence of Yersinia can be tested by a comprehensive stool analysis by requesting Yersinia to be added to the test panel.

Additionally, some viruses, including the Coxsackie virus, hepatitis C virus, HTLV-1 (human T-lymphotropic Virus 1), enterovirus, rubella, mumps, parvovirus and the Epstein-Barr Virus (the virus that causes mono), have been implicated.

Antibodies, which indicate exposure to these viruses, were found to be more prevalent in Hashimoto's patients compared with healthy controls. Interestingly, the Epstein-Barr virus also causes antibodies to T3. This would show up as elevated T3, but low free T3 on lab tests.

Dr. Brownstein reports that he finds underlying infections in many autoimmune illnesses. These underlying infections may be part of the cause of the autoimmune condition. By treating the infections many of the symptoms of the conditions will improve or resolve.

Some organisms that have been identified by Dr. Brownstein in Hashimoto's and in other autoimmune conditions include; Borrelia burgdorferi, Brucella, Candida albicans, Chlamydia, Coxiella, fungi, Hepatitis B, Mycobacterium tuberculosis, Mycoplasma, Neisseria, Parvovirus, Staphylococcus aureus, Streptococcus, Treponema pallidum as well as certain viruses.

Researchers have identified Mycoplasma, Candida, and Epstein-Barr virus as the infections most commonly associated with Hashimoto's.

Hijackers

Bacteria and viruses have a way of modulating our immune system for their own protection, and become "disguised" in our bodies, sending out messages to the immune system that prevent the immune system from destroying them.

Thus a pathogen may be "hiding out" in one of the target organs of an autoimmune attack and damaging the organ and causing inflammation. The inflammation is recognized by the immune system, and the immune system instead attacks the tissue of the organ.

Epstein-Barr is a virus that causes mononucleosis (commonly called "Mono"), a debilitating viral infection that is common among college students, and is also known as the "kissing disease," because individuals are exposed to the virus through saliva of those who are infected.

Specific immune cells known as CD8+ T cells are needed to fight off the Epstein-Barr virus, however, some individuals may have a low baseline level of these types of immune cells. (CD8+ T cells decrease with age, are lower in women, and in the presence of low vitamin D intake). When these fighter cells are low, the Epstein-Barr virus may take up residence in our organs (such as the thyroid) and essentially hijack the organ to help the virus hide and multiply.

Treating Infections

New autoimmune theories have established that once the antigen (trigger) is removed, the antibody production goes away and the innocent part of our bodies (in the case of Hashimoto's, the TPO enzyme) is no longer a target.

As iodine has been identified to be a trigger for Hashimoto's, patients are advised to reduce iodine intake. This will prevent the expression of TPO, which is a "bystander" and gets attacked by the immune system every time that it is released. Iodine restriction will also prevent the iodination of thyroglobulin, making it less likely to be a target of the immune system. For others, adrenal dysfunction is a trigger, and adrenal stressors need to be eliminated in order to allow the body to heal.

In the case of infections, once the infection is removed, the TPO should no longer be a trigger once the immune system recognizes that the infection is gone. Thus, treating infections may help to heal Hashimoto's. In other cases, the infection may be gone and the immune system may need a reboot.

Antibiotics for Autoimmune Conditions

Studies done on mouse models of Type I diabetes mellitus (DM) found that the use of some antibiotics actually prevented the development of Type 1 DM (the antibiotics studied were: fusidic acid, Colistin™, Bactrim™, and doxycycline).

Numerous bacterial agents have also been implicated in triggering the development of Hashimoto's. These agents include: Yersinia enterocolitica, Mycobacterium avium subspecies paratuberculosis (MAP), and H. Pylori. MAP and H. Pylori have also been implicated in Graves' disease, another autoimmune thyroid condition that causes hyperthyroidism (an overactive thyroid). Interestingly, two medications used to treat Graves' disease, thiourea and methimazole have shown antibacterial activity against MAP.

Dr. Brownstein reports that most cases of autoimmune thyroid disorders are caused by infectious agents and tests his patients for hidden infections. He uses pulsed antibiotics such as doxycycline in his treatment plan for autoimmune thyroid conditions when infections are recognized.

Some individuals have reported the normalization of thyroid peroxidase antibodies following taking the antibiotic doxycycline, which is effective for Yersinia enterocolitica as well as other Gram-negative bacteria. Others with Hashimoto's report feeling better after taking doxycycline, antiviral, anti-parasitic, or antifungal medications and herbs.

Work with your doctor to test for infections, and use antibiotics judiciously, as they can be incredibly dangerous when used incorrectly. There is a multitude of different antibiotics, each with a different group of bacteria they target, and each with their own set of side effects.

Blindly taking antibiotics without knowing the cause of your infection may end up inadvertently destroying the beneficial bacteria.

Be sure to supplement with probiotics during courses of antibiotic therapy, but at different times throughout the day so that the beneficial bacteria in the probiotics are not accidentally killed by the antibiotics. Work with your pharmacist to find out the half-life of your antibiotics and to find an optimal time to take probiotics.

Natural Substances that Can Help Overcome Infections

Probiotics
Extra-virgin coconut oil
Whole cloves of garlic
Fermented foods
Glycyrrhizin (Licorice)
Quercetin
N-acetylcysteine
Coenzyme Q10
Turmeric
Oil of oregano

Parasites

Parasites such as worms, flukes, and protozoa have been found in people with Hashimoto's, fibromyalgia, and other autoimmune conditions. Although we usually think of parasites as being more common in Third World countries, surprisingly, they can be found in Americans as well. Dr. Omar Amin, an expert in parasitology, estimates that 1 in 3 Americans has a parasitic infection.

He recommends parasite testing for anyone suffering from increased intestinal permeability, poor digestion, allergies, fatigue, irritable bowel, gas, bloating, cramps, and other gastrointestinal symptoms.

Parasite tests that are available include blood tests (a specific parasite must be requested), fecal tests that look for eggs or parasites, as well as endoscopy/colonoscopy, where a tube is inserted into the intestines to examine the contents.

A comprehensive stool analysis is the most useful test used for finding parasites, but often times tests for specific parasites need to be requested, as they are not included in the standard work-up. The labs will examine the stools for parasites and signs that they may be present (such as eggs). Newer tests use DNA analysis.

There are limitations to the stool test as the parasites may not always be expelled in the stools that are tested. As such, a minimum of three stool tests is recommended by the Centers for Disease Control when parasites are suspected. Additionally, there are many different parasite species that are capable of infecting humans, but often labs test only for a few different species.

A negative test result is not always definitive. Some individuals with autoimmune and other health concerns reported that tests they had were negative for parasites, but they expelled parasites following a parasite cleansing protocol.

Furthermore, not all labs are created equally. Some may be better equipped to handle parasite testing. Dr. Amin runs a lab that is dedicated to comprehensive parasite testing. Additionally, the lab runs testing for other causes of gastrointestinal distress such as candida, bacterial infections and opportunistic bacteria.

Hashimoto's is associated with immune system dysfunction, intestinal permeability, and nutrient depletion. Parasites can shift the immune system and cause intestinal permeability as well as deplete the body of nutrients. As all of these factors seem to be present in Hashimoto's, it may be wise to investigate the role of parasitic infections as a potential trigger for Hashimoto's.

Immune compromise, nutrient deficiencies, low stomach acid, and a lack of beneficial bacteria may make Hashimoto's patients especially susceptible to parasites. Parasites can be picked up from overseas travel, as well as from American soils, waters, meat, and pets.

Symptoms of parasitic infections include intermittent diarrhea and constipation, digestive issues, hemorrhoids, pain with bowel movements, mucous in the stools, gas, bloating, anal itching, and vitamin and mineral deficiencies. Some individuals report insomnia and intolerance to certain foods. However, parasites can also live in our bodies without causing any symptoms.

Medications for parasites are available with a prescription, and those who have discovered a parasite through testing should work with their physicians to take the proper medication.

Natural remedies are available for parasites as well, and some individuals have found that symptoms of their autoimmune conditions improve following natural parasite cleanse products.

Antiparasitic Herbs

Aloe *(Aloe Barbadensis)*
Anise *(Pimpinella Anisum)*
Barberry *(Berberis Vulgaris)*
Black Walnuts *(Juglans Nigra)*
Cashew *(Anacardium Occidentale)*
Curled Mint *(Mentha Crispa)*
Garlic *(Allium Sativum)*
Goldenseal *(Hydrastis Canadensis)*
Grapefruit Seed Extract *(Gynandropis Gynandra)*
Oregon Grape *(Berberis Aquifolium)*
Papaya *(Carica Papaya)*
Pomegranate *(Punica Granatum)*
Pumpkin *(Cucurbitae Semen)*
Sweet Basil *(Ocimum Basilicum)*
Thyme *(Thymus Vulgaris)*
Turmeric *(Curcuma Longa)*
Wormwood *(Artemisia Annua)*

Parasite Cleanse

Simple carbohydrates, refined foods, juices, and dairy as well as fruit can help parasites proliferate, and should be avoided if parasites are suspected.

Substances that have been reported to help with eliminating parasites and can be included in the diet include raw garlic, pumpkin seeds, pomegranates, beets and carrots. Fiber may also help the body clear out worms. Papaya seeds and papaya extracts (papain) have been helpful in eliminating worms and keeping the intestine in a natural acidic state. Probiotics, zinc and vitamin C have also been reported to be helpful by helping to restore immune function.

Certain herbs can also be used to get rid of parasites and can be found in various mixtures and amounts in parasite cleansing formulas such as Humaworm and Freedom/Cleanse/Restore, a formula made by Dr. Amin's clinic. The herbs are not without side effects and should be used with caution, preferably under the supervision of a trained herbalist.

Chapter Summary

- ✓ Autoimmune conditions can be triggered by infections.
- ✓ Many types of infections have been implicated in Hashimoto's.
- ✓ Test for parasitic, bacterial, viral, and fungal infections.
- ✓ People with Hashimoto's are at higher risk for parasitic infections due to impaired digestion.
- ✓ Eliminate infections as needed.

"Your present circumstances don't determine where you can go; they merely determine where you start".- Nido Qubein

10: IMMUNE IMBALANCE

The Chicken or the Egg?

An alternative theory to pathogens causing autoimmunity is that autoimmunity causes an impairment in our ability to keep the pathogens under control, and thus people with autoimmune conditions may test positive for more pathogens than those without autoimmune conditions.

When considering targets for therapy, we always look at systems that are malfunctioning. Scientists look to the immune system imbalance to identify potential opportunities to make an impact on autoimmune conditions.

Immune System Overview

White blood cells (also known as leukocytes) are immune cells that help us defend against foreign invaders and infections. They are produced in the bone marrow and can develop into a few different types of cells including lymphocytes (lymph cells).

Lymphocytes are further differentiated into B cells (these make antibodies that mark pathogens by binding to them to aid in their destruction); Natural Killer Cells (these target infected or cancerous cells), and T cells. T cells are the main cell types implicated in host defense (fighting pathogenic invasions like our friends the CD8+ T cells) and autoimmunity, specifically the T helper (Th) cells.

In response to threats, the immune system is able to decide which types of cells should be produced. All Th cells start as naïve T-helper cells (Thp), and are produced in the bone marrow. They are further differentiated into three different cell types; Th-1 cells are produced in response to bacteria and viruses, Th-2 cells are summoned in response to parasites, and Th-17 cells in response to fungi. Additionally, the thymus produces T regulatory cells, which are responsible for suppressing the immune response and for self-tolerance.

Figure 6: T helper Cell Differentiation

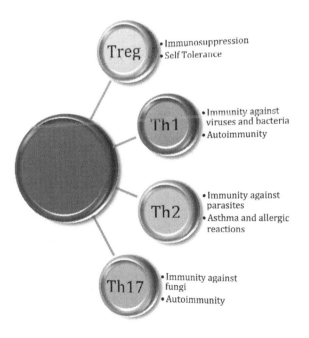

Adapted from Sanna Filén S. Lahesmaa R. GIMAP Proteins in T-Lymphocytes, Journal of Signal Transduction, vol. 2010, 2010.

Each T-cell type produces different interleukins (IL) that act as signaling molecules for various immune processes, and also act as signals to the thymus to send more reinforcements, stimulating more of their own production, and suppressing the production of other cytokines (i.e., Th-1 cytokines stimulate the production of Th-1 cytokines and suppress Th2 cytokines, and vice versa). In normal conditions, a balance of these types of cells is maintained, however, in autoimmune conditions, an imbalance occurs.

Th-1

Th-1 cells are part of the branch of the immune system known as cellular or cell-mediated immunity, and act as our line of defense against intracellular pathogens, or pathogens that live and replicate *inside of our cells,* such as viruses and some types of bacteria. This type of immune response is the most effective in removing virus-infected cells, but also is involved in responses to fungi, protozoans, cancers, and intracellular bacteria through lymphocytes. Cell-mediated immunity is associated with immune rejection of transplanted organs.

Cell-mediated immunity is an immune response that does not produce antibodies but instead activates different types of cells including phagocytes, natural killer cells (NK) and antigen-specific cytotoxic T-lymphocytes to attack and kill virus-infected cells, cells infected with bacteria, and cancer cells. Inadequate Th-1 response has been associated with chronic infections and cancer.

This arm of the immune system produces TNF alpha, interferon (INF) gamma, IL-2, and IL-12, which stimulate natural killer cells and cytotoxic cells and are pro-inflammatory. The Th-1 Immune Response is associated with inflammation and delayed type hypersensitivity as well as IgG2 antibodies, like the ones produced in Hashimoto's. An increase in Th-1 cells has been found in Hashimoto's, and a prominent increase is seen in more severe cases.

Certain immune modulating medications based on the naturally occurring Th-1 substances, including interferon (used to treat hepatitis) and IL-2, (used to treat melanoma) have been associated with Hashimoto's Thyroiditis development. These medications/cytokines suppress T-regulatory calls and shift to the production of Th-1 cells.

Th-2 cells

The Th-2 pathway is known as humoral mediated immunity. It is named this way because it involves extracellular substances, or the substances found *outside of our cells,* in body fluids (humorous).

This pathway becomes activated in the presence of parasites that invade the areas surrounding our cells, such as worms. The cytokines produced by this pathway are: IL-4, IL-5, IL-9, IL-13. These cytokines suppress the production of the Th-1 inflammatory cytokines and stimulate the production of B cells. The B cells are responsible for the production of antibodies to mark the invaders and direct the immune response.

An overactive Th-2 system has been implicated in IgE mediated allergic reactions such as the very annoying seasonal pollen allergies, as well as the life-threatening anaphylactic reactions to bee stings, shellfish, and nuts.

Th-17

Th-17 cells have recently been implicated in autoimmune conditions. Th-17 cells become activated in the presence of extracellular microbes, or microbes that live outside of our cells such as fungi and some bacteria.

These cells produce IL-17, IL-23 which are pro-inflammatory

cytokines active against Citrobacter, Klebsiella pneumoniae, and Candida albicans pathogenic species, and can initiate autoimmunity.

IL-17a is pro-inflammatory cytokine and causes direct toxicity to the cells it encounters. Th-17 activation has been implicated in both Hashimoto's and Graves'.

T regulatory cells

T regulatory cells (Tregs) are formerly known as suppressor T cells, and their role is to return the immune system to balance after an infection. They are produced in the thymus and have anti-inflammatory and immunosuppressive actions as well as promote the immune tolerance of self. Tregs are associated with the immunosuppressive cytokines: TGF-Beta and IL-10. Tregs seem to have an inverse relationship with Th-17 cells, meaning the more Th-17 cells present, the fewer cells will be differentiated into Tregs. A reduction of Treg cells has been found in autoimmune conditions including Hashimoto's, while an increase has been found in cancers and infections that trick the body to increase Treg production so they can blend in unnoticed by the immune system. Mouse models have shown that depletion of Tregs leads to hypothyroidism.

Immune Imbalance

In normal conditions, the immune branches work together to overcome an infection. A healthy immune system is able to balance among each of these branches, and rapidly shift the balance to the types of cells that are needed most when we are battling an infection. It is also able to turn off the production of the fighter cells when they are no longer needed. An imbalance of any of these branches results in autoimmune conditions, or a lack of self-recognition.

Thus an immune "imbalance" has been proposed in most

autoimmune conditions. For example, an increased number of Th-1 cells has been associated with Hashimoto's, while an increased number of Th-2 cells has been associated with Graves' disease and asthma.

However, this is not the case for all people affected, and some people with Hashimoto's may have an overabundance of Th-2 cells or not have a clear predominating pathway.

An overabundance of inflammatory cytokines resulting from the Th-1, Th-2, and/or Th-17 system, in relation to not enough immune suppressive cytokines produced by Tregs, is usually associated with autoimmune conditions.

Stress, pregnancy, and hormonal imbalances may be associated with shifting the immune balance (more info on hormonal balance can be found in the "Triggers" chapter).

Insufficiency of adrenal hormones can also shift the body into Th-1 dominance. As our adrenal hormones become depleted during times of stress, it is therefore not surprising that the development of autoimmunity has often been linked with periods of extreme and/or prolonged chronic stress. The significance of the adrenals and stress in the development of Hashimoto's will be discussed in the "Adrenals" chapter.

The Th-2 branch of the immune system may also become overactive in the presence of insulin surges (that lead to increase B-cell production).

Many autoimmune conditions are associated with an over-representation of cells being differentiated to Th-2 cells (antibody production). Women, who represent 90% of those affected with autoimmune conditions, generally present a predominant Th-2 cytokine profile. Hashimoto's seems to be associated with a predominant Th-1 cytokine differentiation. In his book, "Why Am I still Having Thyroid Symptoms When my Lab Tests are Normal?", Dr. Datis Kharrazian states that Hashimoto's patients may be afflicted with either type of imbalance, but the majority present with a Th-1 dominance.

Cellular Immunity Mediated (Th-1)	Humoral Immunity Mediated (Th-2)
Hashimoto's thyroiditis	Graves' disease
Multiple sclerosis	Asthma
Rheumatoid arthritis	Lupus
Crohn's disease	Seasonal allergies
Type 1 diabetes	Ulcerative colitis
Psoriasis	
Giant papillary conjunctivitis	

Studies have found that Hashimoto's patients have an increased amount of Th-1 cells that produce Interferon Gamma, which promotes inflammation, as well as more IL-2, IL-12 and IL-18, which are also cytokines produced by the Th-1 cells. Additionally, a decreased amount of Th-2-produced IL-4 was found, which is protective against autoimmune inflammatory disease.

Table 9: Cytokines in Hashimoto's :

Cytokine	Hashimoto's	Healthy Controls	Statistically Significant?
IL-2	12.16 ± 0.66	7.36 ± 0.45	Yes
IFN-G	7.6 ± 0.33	5.09 ± 0.27	Yes
IL-12	3.57 ± 0.19	2.59 ± 0.23	Yes
IL-18	27.52 ± 1.75	15.16 ± 1.62	Yes

Adapted from: Phenekos C, et. al. Th1 and Th2 serum cytokine profiles characterize patients with Hashimoto's thyroiditis (Th1) and Graves' disease (Th2). Neuroimmunomodulation. 2004;11(4):209-13

Th-17 cells were found in both autoimmune thyroid conditions.

Th-1 and Th-17 were both found in thyroid cells in mice with Hashimoto's, and it is proposed that IL-17 cells are critical for the development of Hashimoto's. New research suggests that Th-17 rather than Th-1 may be causing the damage involved in the pathogenesis of Hashimoto's. This would explain why some Hashimoto patients present with a mix of Th-1 and Th-2 dominance, and also with no clearly defined dominance.

Immune Modulating Substances

Some natural substances have been shown to shift our immune system to produce more Th-1 cells, such as beta-glucan mushrooms, Echinacea, and licorice root. These products are sometimes advertised as "immune boosters" or "immune stimulants." Additionally, low-intensity exercises like walking, tai chi, and restorative yoga, the probiotic strain Lactobacillus plantarum and Gyokuheifusan, an herbal formula in traditional Chinese medicine, has also been shown to support the production of Th-1 type cells in clinical trials.

In contrast, substances like pine bark extract, curcumin from turmeric, green tea, and resveratrol have been shown to drive the production of Th-2 type cells. Workouts that are higher intensity and of longer duration have also been reported to increase the Th-2 response.

When one arm of the immune system is overactive, balance may be restored through using substances that strengthen the underactive arm or weaken the overactive arm.

While many will agree that the Th-1/Th-2 ratio may be "imbalanced" in autoimmune conditions, blindly trying to manipulate the balance may be detrimental. One must know which side of the scale is down to restore balance.

Table 10: Immune Modulating Substances

Stimulate Th-1 cell production	Stimulate Th-2 cell production
Ashwaganda	Alcohol
Astragalus	Anatabine
Beta-glucan mushrooms and other immune boosting mushrooms	Candida
Chlorella and other algae products*	Candida
Echinacea	Cortisol
Estrogen	Curcumin from turmeric
Glutathione	DHEA
Gram-negative bacteria (endotoxin)	Genistein
Licorice root	Green tea extract
Melissa officinalis (lemon balm)	Lycopene
Panax ginseng	Parasites
Polypodium leucotomos fern extract (Difur)	Pine bark extract
Selenium	Pycnogenol (natural ingredient in apples)
Viruses	Quercetin
Yoga, restorative exercise	Resveratrol
	Soluble fiber
	Vigorous exercise
	White willow bark

*Algae may contain high amounts of iodine

Acupuncture

Acupuncture has been reported to balance the Th-1/Th-2 ratio and has been found to be helpful in a variety of conditions including infertility, endometriosis, and pain, as well as autoimmune conditions. Acupuncture is thought to cause physical responses in nerve cells promoting the release of cytokines that regulate the immune system. Recent studies have demonstrated that acupuncture can help rebalance Th-1 disorders by promoting Th-2 cytokines, and was helpful in Type IV Hypersensitivity reactions, like Hashimoto's. For those who are skeptical and cite the "placebo effect," it is noteworthy to learn that in addition to patient reports, many of these studies were done in animals such as dogs, rats, and guinea pigs.

Personally, my TPO antibodies fell from the 2,000 range to the mid-300s after receiving acupuncture. My antibodies remained low for over a year but started to creep up after stopping acupuncture when I moved to a different state.

Cytokine Testing and Cytokine Ratios

Cytokine tests can be ordered by doctors and patients alike to check to see which branch of the immune system is overactive.

One may be able to measure the cytokines at baseline and follow up with re-testing after an intervention is made. As a word of caution, these labs are considered "for research purposes only," and are not recognized to aid or cure any disease, thus they are not usually covered by insurance companies.

In these labs the various cytokines expressed by the Th-1 and Th-2 branches are measured.

As an alternate, some practitioners recommend testing out one or more of the substances associated with strengthening either the Th-1 or Th-2 arm. The theory is that if one takes a Th-1 strengthening substance and feels better, she must have an overactive Th-2 system, while if she feels worse, she will have an overactive Th-1 system, and vice versa. Symptoms to watch for may include: heart palpitations, anxiety, trembling, insomnia, irritability and/or excessive sweating. These are signs of *hyperthyroidism* and occur when too much thyroid hormone is rapidly dumped into circulation as a result of increasing thyroid destruction.

While some may feel their condition getting better or worse after such as test, I personally feel that many of us may need an objective measure to define worsening or improvement of our condition.

Some professionals are proposing taking a mix of a multitude of various supplements to try to shift one's Th-1/Th-2 balance. This may be helpful for some, but not for all of those with Hashimoto's.

Furthermore, while taking supplements on a chronic basis to "dim" the immune response may be helpful for treating *symptoms;* it does not get to the *root cause* of Hashimoto's.

Additionally, Th-17 cells have been found to be present in most cases of autoimmune conditions, and they seem to suppress the production of Treg cells.

Researchers are now suggesting that immune modulation should be **anti-inflammatory** and aimed at increasing the production of more **T-regulatory cells**, not on trying to manipulate the Th-1/Th-2 ratio. An increased amount of Tregs should rebalance the Th-1/Th-2 ratio through suppression and promotion of recognition and tolerance of self-antigens by down-regulating an overactive immune system.

Anti-Inflammatory Approach

In doing research for healing myself, I found that smoking tobacco reduces the risk of Hashimoto's. This angered me because here I was a former smoker trying to be more healthy and instead I get stuck with an autoimmune condition. Of course starting to smoke again would be foolish because of the many other risks that greatly outweigh the benefits. I wondered what about smoking reduced the incidence of Hashimoto's, until I came across a new supplement.

Anatabine

Anatabine is a naturally occurring alkaloid found in the Nightshade plant family (tomato, tobacco, peppers) that is available as a dietary supplement. Anatabine has anti-inflammatory effects and reduces the expression of cytokines (IL-18, IL-1R2) associated with the development of Th-1 mediated autoimmunity.

Researchers from John Hopkins have shown that anatabine reduced the incidence and severity of Hashimoto's in mice.

Clinical trials have recently been completed with humans and showed a significant reduction in TPO antibodies, as well as a decrease in inflammation over a period of three months. The data from the trials is not available at the time of writing this book, however, the manufacturer has provided a few case examples.

One patient who was studied had an enormous drop in antibody levels after she took a dose of 0.12 mg/kg per day of anatabine for sixteen days. Her TPO antibodies reduced from 3655 IU to 300 IU.

Doses of 0.12 mg/kg per day to 0.267mg/kg per day have been studied and found to be safe and effective in reducing TPO antibodies. This dose would equal to about 5 mg–12 mg per day for a 100-pound woman. Anatabine has a half-life of about eight hours, and should be dosed six to eight hours apart to ensure a constant level in the body.

Anatabine should be started at a low dose of 1–2 mg per day and gradually increased to the target dose over a week. The onset of action should be seen within a couple of days to a few weeks. Early research suggests that anatabine must be taken continuously to exert its effect on the immune system.

Side effects of headache, nausea, vomiting, and changes in liver function have been observed when doses were started too high.

This supplement may be a helpful tool in reducing inflammation and antibodies while searching for why the immune system is imbalanced.

Note: some individuals with Hashimoto's may have a nightshade sensitivity.

Curcumin

Curcumin, from the spice turmeric, has anti-inflammatory benefits that can be helpful in down-regulating autoimmune conditions. Curcumin produces an anti-inflammatory effect by down-regulating Th-1 cytokines (TNF-A, IL-1, 2, 6, 8, 12).

Curcumin has been found to reduce joint inflammation in the Th-1 autoimmune condition rheumatoid arthritis. Additionally, it seems to have therapeutic anti-inflammatory effects in a variety of gastrointestinal conditions. Curcumin improved Crohn's disease (Th-1), Ulcerative colitis (Th-2) and IBS.

Although some researchers suggested that the daily intake of curcumin in a typical Indian diet may be anti-inflammatory, the amount of curcumin present in spices may not enough to produce anti-inflammatory benefits for autoimmune conditions. Curcumin may be taken as a supplement, but by itself it is quickly excreted out of the body, and thus needs to be combined with peperine, an alkaloid found in pepper, to be remain active for a longer time in the body.

Curcumin appears to be extremely safe, even at doses of up to 8 grams/day, however, some individuals with Hashimoto's (especially those with Nightshade sensitivities) may have an intolerance to peperine and may not be able to use the supplement.

Increasing Regulatory T-Cells

Autoimmune conditions are also more likely to cluster in regions farther from equator. This is likely because of inadequate vitamin D levels. Vitamin D deficiency is associated with improper immune function—a lack of CD8+ T cells that kill off viruses like EBV and a lack of T-regulatory cells that keep the immune system balanced.

In recent years, the role of vitamin D in the health of human body has been strongly emphasized by researchers and the medical community alike. Serum vitamin D levels can be directly correlated with human life expectancy. Dr. William Grant, Ph.D., a vitamin D expert, has proposed that raising the serum vitamin D level would prevent 30% of cancer deaths each year.

Vitamin D affects about 3,000–30,000 genes in our bodies, and many diseases have also been connected to vitamin D levels, including heart disease, depression, and autoimmune conditions.

Vitamin D is known for its role in balancing Th-1 (cell-mediated) and Th-2 (humoral) immune system responses by influencing T-regulatory (Treg) cells, which are responsible for the control, expression and differentiation of Th-1 and Th-2.

Vitamin D actively prevents the development of autoimmunity in animal models, and there is strong connection between vitamin D deficiency and autoimmune thyroiditis.

In humans, serum levels of 1,25(OH) 2D3 were found to be significantly lower in autoimmune than non-autoimmune hyperthyroidism.

As skin cancer awareness and the use of sunscreen has become more widespread, people are not getting the appropriate amount of vitamin

D in the summertime, and those living in northern climates are especially at risk for vitamin D deficiency in the colder months.

Vitamin D deficiency is one of the most under-recognized deficiencies in our society and an estimated 85% of Americans may be deficient. A study in Turkey found that 92% of Hashimoto's patients were deficient in vitamin D. Studies are now suggesting that much higher doses of vitamin D than the current RDA of 400 IU per day should be taken.

Testing for Vitamin D Deficiency

If you live in a northern climate and don't spend time outside on a daily basis, you are at risk for vitamin D deficiency.

Vitamin D levels should be between **60 and 80 ng/L** for optimal thyroid receptor and immune system function. Vitamin D levels should be checked at regular intervals, especially in the winter seasons. There are two available tests: 1,25 (OH)D and 25(OH)D. The test 25(OH)D, also called 25-hydroxyl vitamin D, is preferred.

Sources of vitamin D include: cod liver oil, fish, fortified dairy and orange juice, eggs, and most importantly, sunlight. In fact, the farther we get from the equator, the higher our likelihood of developing an autoimmune condition.

We may be tempted to eat more foods with vitamin D in an effort to be natural and healthy. However, the amount of vitamin D in foods may not do the job for everyone.

People with Graves' disease, another autoimmune thyroid condition, have been found to have altered binding of vitamin D, while abnormalities in vitamin D receptor genes have been found in many other autoimmune conditions. These individuals have trouble converting supplemental vitamin D to its active form. Additionally, EBV and other pathogens can hijack the vitamin D receptor, rendering vitamin D supplements useless.

Your Prescription? A Beach Vacation!

The best way to restore optimal vitamin D level is through sun exposure, safe tanning beds, and an oral vitamin D3 supplement. The best sources of vitamin D from food come from wild salmon, 800 IU/3.5 oz of D3; and cod liver oil, 700 IU per teaspoon.

What can we learn from bacteria and parasites?

Research has found that some types of bacteria actively manipulate regulatory T cells to help their own survival in the host. Certain probiotic strains have been used in mouse models of autoimmune disease and have been found to increase T cell differentiation to produce more Tregs and had an impact on disease outcomes (arthritis, asthma). These beneficial bacterial strains included (L. casei, L. salivarius, lacotobacillus rhamnosus, bifidobacterium lactis, l. reuteri). Another study was done with lactobacillus plantarum, which was responsible for reducing the risk for anaphylactic type of allergies by increasing the Th-1 response.

In contrast, in vitro studies (in lab conditions), showed that Bifidobacterium bifidum and lactobacillus acidophilus were actually found to block the suppressive activities of Tregs, while Bifidobacterium animalis produced more inflammation. So buyer beware—not all probiotics are created equally. Some may be beneficial to certain autoimmune conditions while others not.

In addition to probiotics, which will be further discussed in subsequent chapters, other ways of increasing T-regulatory cells have been identified, including such activities as weightlifting and sunbathing in ultraviolet light, as well as foods and supplements.

Substances that have been found to increase the amount of T-regs
EGCG, a compound found in green tea
Weightlifting
Bone marrow manipulation
Ultraviolet light
Vitamin A
Vitamin D
Papaya
Butyrate
L-glutathione
Superoxide dismutase

Certain substances have been reported to weaken the immune system, and should be removed from our diets. They include processed foods, pro-inflammatory vegetable oils, white sugar, and alcohol.

Conditions such as leaky gut, low hydrochloric acid, and poor digestion, which result in circulating immune complexes (CICs); low body temperature, exposure to heavy metals and environmental pollutants, tobacco smoke, presence of viral, bacterial, or fungal pathogens also weaken the immune system and should be addressed.

Lifestyle factors like a sedentary lifestyle, negative attitudes, chronic stress, insomnia, and rapid muscle building (with heavy weightlifting or anabolic steroids) have also contributed to a weakened immune system and should be modified to ensure a healthy immune function. In contrast, immune strengthening substances that have been identified include: garlic extract (also has antimicrobial function), vitamin E (an antioxidant), ginkgo biloba (through reduction of excess cortisol production), colostrum, DHEA (an adrenal hormone), olive oil, coconut oil, the herb neem, vitamin A, cod liver oil, L-glutamine, probiotics, low-dose Naltrexone (LDN), and omega-3 fatty acids.

Adequate hydration, exercise, meditation, a positive outlook, forgiveness, letting go of resentments, and long-term goals are also beneficial not just to our overall well-being but also to immune function.

Low-Dose Naltrexone

Low-Dose Naltrexone (LDN) has been reported to enhance immune function through increasing our endogenous adrenaline production, reducing inflammatory cytokines, promoting DNA synthesis, and slowing down motility in the GI tract to facilitate healing. LDN increases the amount of T-regulatory cytokines IL-1 and TGF-B, leading to a reduction of Th-17, the promoter of autoimmunity.

Naltrexone is an FDA-approved medication used for opioid withdrawal at a dose of 50 mg per day. However, only low doses of 1.5–4.5 mg per day have been found to tweak the immune system and have shown promise in improving cases of autoimmune disease, including Crohn's, MS and Hashimoto's, as well as other immune system-related conditions such as cancer and HIV/AIDS.

The website dedicated to sharing research on LDN, www.lowdosenaltrexone.org, is full of testimonials about ulcers, tumors, and lesions disappearing within months of initiating LDN.

The authors of the website even caution users with Hashimoto's taking supplemental thyroid hormone to start low (1.5 mg per night) and watch for emerging signs of hyperthyroidism that may result from rapid improvement of the condition.

This medication is available only as a prescription and can be compounded into lower doses by special professional compounding pharmacies (or a resourceful person with a mortar and pestle and precise measuring tools). Luckily, even without insurance coverage, this medication is available in generic form and is very affordable.

I have tried low-dose Naltrexone, but found that it made me somewhat irritable after a few nights of taking it. However, this was before I started working on my diet, and I have since heard anecdotal evidence of LDN working best when used in combination with a leaky gut diet.

Chapter Summary

✓ An immune system imbalance is present in Hashimoto's, which results in more inflammation.

✓ Vitamin D deficiency is connected to autoimmunity. Measure levels of vitamin D.

✓ Increase vitamin D via beach vacationing, tanning, or vitamin D supplements/food to get vitamin D levels between 60 and 80 ng/ml.

✓ Antabine is a supplement that has been shown to reduce TPO antibodies by preventing an inflammatory reaction.

✓ Curcumin with peperine has shown promise in reducing inflammatory autoimmune responses and gut inflammation.

✓ Low-dose Naltrexone is a prescription medication that modulates the immune system to reduce the autoimmune attack.

✓ Immune-modulating substances may be helpful in slowing down or halting thyroid cell destruction while we work to identify and eliminate triggers and fix intestinal permeability.

11: THE GUT

So the big question is ... how to we restore our health and our immune system? And it seems all roads lead back to Rome!

While various pathogens have been found to be associated with Hashimoto's, researchers are not able to establish a definite causal link between any specific pathogens and Hashimoto's. This means that not everyone with these infections, even having the genetic susceptibility, develops Hashimoto's. Additionally, not everyone with Hashimoto's has these infections. Other potential triggers have also been identified in Hashimoto's and include iodine, stress, toxins, and our internal microbial flora.

In addition to the genetic susceptibility and the triggers, there is a third piece of the puzzle that must be present for Hashimoto's to develop.

This common link is present in all autoimmune conditions, and gets closer to the root cause of the development of autoimmunity: Increased intestinal permeability a.k.a. "leaky gut."

So what does the gut have to do with the immune system and autoimmunity? Everything! It is the intestinal lining that prevents autoimmunity!

Researchers have found that in addition to digesting and absorbing nutrients, and keeping a water and electrolyte balance, the intestine is also responsible for helping the immune system recognize foreign invaders from self-antigens, thus facilitating the control of pathogens and preventing autoimmune reactions.

Intestinal Wall

A layer of epithelial cells covers the entire intestine and has the important role of keeping a protective mucosal barrier between the dirty environment inside of our intestines (partially digested food, pollens, feces, dead cells, bacteria, etc.) and the rest of our body where those substances could do potential harm.

This layer is formed by intercellular tight junctions analogous to thread fibers that make up a piece of cloth. These threads, however, are not static and their proximity to one another or "tightness" can be affected by various factors.

What Exactly is "Leaky Gut"?

"Leaky gut" is an abnormally increased permeability of the small intestine. In leaky gut, the intestinal tight junctions become looser, allowing substances that normally would not gain systemic access to get into the circulation.

Once substances like food, bacteria and self-antigens get past the intestinal barrier into the circulation, the immune system recognizes them as foreign substances, which leads to inflammation in the body and gut, further increasing permeability and triggering food sensitivities and autoimmunity.

What Causes Leaky Gut?

Dr. Fasano has identified that in the presence of leaky gut, we secrete excess zonulin, a protein that modulates the permeability between the tight junctions. An excess of this protein has been found in virtually every autoimmune condition! A variety of factors has been implicated in causing an excess release of this protein, and include gliadin (gluten), food intolerances, psychological stress, unsaturated fats, non-steroidal anti-inflammatory drugs (NSAIDs) like Advil™ and Aleve™, alcohol, pathogenic bacteria, as well as an overgrowth of bacteria from the large intestine (colon) into the small intestine. This increased permeability is thought to be a defensive mechanism for clearing bacteria and toxins from the small intestine.

Intestinal permeability can also be increased by various foods and supplements as well as surgery, trauma, and inflammation.

AGES (advanced glycation end products) that are generated from browning or caramelizing foods may also promote inflammation, and can potentially increase intestinal permeability.

Factors that increase intestinal permeability

- Advanced age
- AGES (Advanced Glycation End Products)
- Alcohol
- Capsaicin (sweet peppers, cayenne peppers, paprika)
- Food allergies
- Gliadin (Gluten)
- L-alanine
- Large amounts of tryptophan
- Linoleic acid
- Marigold, hops
- NSAIDs
- Overgrowth of bacteria in small intestine
- Pathogenic bacteria
- Psychological stress (anger, fear)
- Strenuous exercise
- Surgery/Trauma
- Unsaturated fats
- Zonulin

Intestinal Tight Junctions

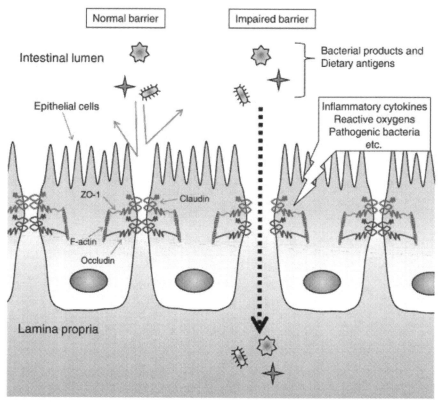

Figure 7: Intestinal epithelial Tight Junctions (TJs) act as a physical barrier. The intestinal TJs tightly regulate intestinal permeability. The barrier impairment allows bacterial products and dietary antigens to cross the epithelium and enter circulation. This can induce inflammation and immunological reactions in tissues including the intestines, resulting in both intestinal and autoimmune diseases.

Figure reprinted from The Journal of Nutritional Biochemistry Vol. 22, Suzuki, T. Hara, H . Role of flavonoids in intestinal tight junction regulation. Fig 1. Copyright 2011. Reprinted with permission from Elsevier.

TESTING FOR INTESTINAL PERMEABILITY

Testing for intestinal permeability is fairly simple and non-invasive through the Mannitol-Lactulose Intestinal Permeability Test.

The patient drinks a premeasured amount of two sugars: lactulose and mannitol. The degree of intestinal permeability or malabsorption is reflected in the levels of the two sugars recovered in a urine sample collected over the next six hours.

Mannitol, a monosaccharide, should be well absorbed by the intestinal barrier. In contrast, lactulose, a disaccharide, is normally not absorbed unless the intestinal barrier is compromised.

The test measures the ration of lactulose to mannitol in the urine. An elevated ratio means that excessive lactulose was absorbed, indicating leaky gut syndrome.

Tests can be repeated to gauge progress with leaky gut treatment.

PILLARS OF OPTIMAL GUT FUNCTION

In order to fix our immune system, we must restore optimal gut function. The pillars of optimal gut function are digestion, elimination, microflora balance, and gut integrity.

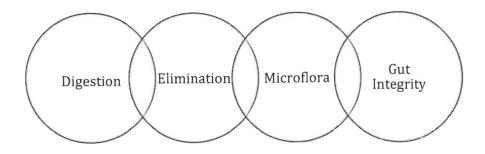

Figure 8: Pillars of Optimal Gut Function

Gut Quiz: Do You Have Symptoms of Impaired Gut Function?

Many people with Hashimoto's and other autoimmune conditions do not immediately associate poor gut function with their immune status. Some may not realize they are having symptoms until they eliminate foods (see the "Intolerances" chapter).

- ☐ I have a bloated or full feeling, and/or belching, burning, or flatulence right after meals.
- ☐ I have chronic yeast or fungal infections.
- ☐ I feel nauseated after taking supplements.
- ☐ I feel fatigued after eating.
- ☐ I have heartburn.
- ☐ I regularly use antacids.
- ☐ I have chronic abdominal pains.
- ☐ I have diarrhea.
- ☐ I have mucous in my bowel movements.
- ☐ I have constipation (going less than once or twice a day).
- ☐ I have greasy, large, poorly formed, or foul-smelling stools.
- ☐ I find food that is not fully digested in my stool.
- ☐ I have food allergies, intolerance, or reactions.
- ☐ I have an intolerance to carbohydrates (eating bread or other sugars causes bloating).
- ☐ I have anal itching.
- ☐ I have bleeding gums or gingivitis.
- ☐ I have geographic tongue (map-like rash on tongue indicating food allergy or yeast overgrowth).
- ☐ I have sores on the tongue.
- ☐ I have canker sores.
- ☐ I crave sweets and bread.

Adapted from Hyman, M., The Ultra Mind Companion Guide. 2009

GUT BACTERIA AT THE ROOT CAUSE OF AUTOIMMUNITY?

When the intestinal lining becomes compromised, gut bacteria that would not otherwise cross the intestinal barrier enter the circulation and cause inflammation. It is also gut bacteria that damage the intestinal lining!

Your gut is home to 100 trillion bacteria, yeasts, and other microbes. You actually have ten times more microbial cells compared with your own cells. Emerging research has shown that the microbial balance in our intestines determines our digestion, immune system balance, emotions, gene expression and overall health status!

Bacterial Universe

Trillions of bacteria live in our intestines in an ever-evolving universe. In fact, the intestinal tract of most adults has anywhere from 300–500 unique bacterial species, many of which have not yet been identified.

Of those species, about thirty to forty species will be the predominant type and account for 99% of the total population. Every individual's bacterial universe has been suggested to be unique, like a fingerprint. As these bacteria are excreted in the feces, predominant species can be measured in the stools of individuals.

The number and types of bacteria also vary throughout the whole intestinal tract. Under normal conditions, the small intestine, the upper part of the GI tract, hosts only a few species of bacteria and has a low number of microorganisms compared with the colon, which has the greatest amount of microorganisms.

Role of Beneficial Bacteria in the Gut

It is our unique resident bacteria that aid with the development of our immune system and determine the type of immune response that should be initiated.

We have all heard of the normal flora, also known as "friendly," "commensal," or "beneficial" bacteria that live in our body in a cooperative environment that benefits their human hosts and the bacteria themselves.

These bacteria utilize the resources provided by the body, such as foods and a comfortable environment for reproduction, and in return provide us with benefits. They help us with the breakdown of non-digested/indigestible foods like polysaccharides; help with the synthesis of micronutrients, short chain fatty acids, and the absorption of trace elements.

The bacteria feed on fiber that is poorly digested by all humans by fermenting it. During the fermentation process, short chain fatty acids, lactate, succinate, ethanol, hydrogen, and carbon dioxide gases are produced.

These beneficial bacteria attach to the intestinal tissue and colonize the gastrointestinal tract. They compete with pathogenic bacteria for intestinal attachment and nutrients and produce substances that kill foreign bacteria and organisms.

This type of arrangement is called a symbiotic relationship, where both the host and bacteria thrive.

Having a good amount of these bacteria helps us metabolize complex carbohydrates, maintain a proper intestinal barrier, and suppress intestinal inflammation.

The best-known beneficial bacteria are from the Lactobacillus and Bifidobacterium species and are classified as Gram-positive bacteria by microbiologists.

Opportunistic Bacteria

Our intestines are also home to other types of bacteria that are known as opportunistic pathogens as they behave well when everything is balanced, but can become naughty when the opportunity arises. These bacteria can become potential pathogens when we are vulnerable, such as in situations of a compromised immune system, impaired digestion, intestinal permeability, depletion of Lactobacillus or Bifidobacterium, and even when we experience psychological stress.

Opportunistic Gram-Negative Bacteria in the Human GI Tract

Hafnia alvei
Pseudomonas aeruginosa
Morganella morganii
Proteus mirabilis
Proteus vulgaris
Pseudomonas putida
Citrobacter koseri
Klebsiella pneumonia

Some of the bacteria in each person's GI tract can be pathogenic when the mucous barrier is compromised.

Dr. Michael Maes is a psychiatrist and pioneer who specializes in treating chronic fatigue syndrome. He has detected increased intestinal permeability in the chronic fatigue patients in his clinic

Dr. Maes and colleagues have found that in the presence of leaky gut, certain Gram-negative enterobacteria that normally reside in human intestines move through the intestinal wall into the circulation in patients with chronic fatigue syndrome and depression.

IgM and IgA antibodies to bacteria normally present in the gut can be detected in the serum when the bacteria cross the intestinal wall into the bloodstream or lymphatic system (bacterial translocation), where they are recognized and attacked by white blood cells.

Through the use of antibody serum tests, Dr. Maes has measured an increased response to endotoxin, a substance that is released by the Gram-negative bacteria in his patients with CFS and depression. He has been able to correlate the patients' symptoms with the levels of IgA and IgM response to endotoxin, thus showing that higher responses to the bacteria translated to more debilitating symptoms of chronic fatigue and depression.

When they gain access to the bloodstream or lymphatic system, the bacteria may act as superantigens or may induce autoimmunity through molecular mimicry

Dysbiosis

Gram-negative enterobacteria are part of the normal flora but become pathogenic under the right circumstances, leading to autoimmunity.

Different bacterial species that are present may produce their own unique byproducts, for example, methanogenic bacteria will produce methane gas during fermentation (not thought to be harmful, unless it is present in excessive amounts when it can cause constipation and IBS), while sulfate-reducing bacteria will produce a harmful hydrogen sulfide gas, which can damage the colonic epithelium.

These gram-negative bacteria are normally present in small amounts in the human intestine, however, some individuals may have too many of them, and not enough of the beneficial gram positive bacteria - this produces an imbalance in bacterial gut flora and is known as gut dysbiosis.

When they predominate, the gram-negative bacteria are able to attach to the intestinal wall and hijack the intestinal barrier, allowing themselves to cross into the blood-stream and lymphatic system.

<u>Proteus bacteria</u>

When there is depletion in beneficial bacteria coupled with poor stomach acid and inadequate protein digestion, the Proteus species of Gram-negative bacteria can overgrow and attach to the intestinal lining. This bacterium damages the cells in the intestinal lining by the toxins it releases when it feeds on partially digested foods though fermenting them. This causes inflammation, leading to an immune system imbalance.

Proteus bacteria do not ferment dairy, but instead ferment fructose and undigested meat. When meat and protein is fermented, this leads to a release of a sulfate gas that damages the intestinal wall. Bad news for those around you: this gas has a rotten-egg smell.

The bacteria then are able to cross into circulation and are implicated in autoimmunity, as the proteins in the cell walls of these bacteria resemble different parts of our self-antigens, thus leading to molecular mimicry. The Proteus bacteria contain lipopolysaccharide (LPS), a type of endotoxin, in their bacterial cell wall. The LPS is released during bacterial death or replication, causing inflammation. As a result, LPS becomes a trigger for the immune system.

Proteus bacterium also liquefies casein, causing it to leak through the intestinal walls and resulting in an immune reaction to casein. Proteus species bacteria have been implicated in causing rheumatoid arthritis through molecular mimicry, as their cell walls look similar to our internal tissues.

Candida

Candida albicans, while not a bacterium, is an opportunistic yeast that is normally present in our intestines, but can become infectious or pathogenic when there is a depletion of beneficial bacteria, nutrients, or a compromised immune system. A history of antibiotics, steroids, pregnancy, recurrent vaginal yeast infections, birth control pills, and a diet rich in simple carbohydrates increases the risk of Candida overgrowth.

Candida overgrowth is present in most people with Hashimoto's. Candida loves starchy foods, sugar, and alcohol. If you too, share this common love with Candida, you may inadvertently end up with an excess candida growth in your intestines.

The symptoms of a candida infection can mimic many of the symptoms of hypothyroidism, including feeling spacey, having cold extremities, and lethargy.

Candida can be controlled by diet, probiotics, supplements, and anti-fungal herbs and medications.

Candida diet: cutting out simple carbohydrates in addition to nuts, seeds, grains, corn, mushrooms, potatoes, fruit, dairy and alcohol is generally recommended to starve the fungus. Ketogenic diets, however, can continue to feed the Candida. (See Diet Chapter).

Candida exists in two forms: the normal yeast spheres and an elongated pathogenic hyphae form. The hyphae form allows Candida to penetrate into the mucosal lining and is responsible for intestinal permeability. Several supplements have been shown to either prevent conversion to the hyphae form or convert it back to its yeast form where it is no longer pathogenic.

These include biotin, thymol (from thyme), carvacrol (from oregano), Eugenol (from cloves), caprylic and undecylenic acid.

Biotin may be especially beneficial for Hashimoto's patients as it is helpful with adrenal function and hair loss. I recommend 5,000 mcg per day.

While most cases of Candida can be controlled with diet and supplements, some cases may require the use of antifungal herbs and even antifungal medications like Nystatin and Fluconazole.

Many books have been written on the subject of overcoming Candida, I recommend The Body Ecology Diet, which is a wonderful resource for those who would like to get additional information.

What Determines the Bacterial Balance?

When we are born, our gut is sterile and we receive most of our bacteria from our mothers. The use of medications, the infections we have had, the types of foods we eat, as well as psychological or physiological stress can promote the proliferation of one type of bacteria while causing another species' populations to diminish.

Medications

Prescriptions and over-the-counter medications that reduce acidity in the small intestine can lead to an overgrowth of bad bacteria. Examples include acid suppressants such as Tums™, Alka-Seltzer™, Pepcid™, and Prilosec™.

Antibiotics can wipe out our normal "protective" flora, allowing pathogenic bacteria to take over. This is because antibiotics often have a "broad spectrum" of activity, which means they are not guided by "GPS" to kill only the pathogenic bacteria, but also kill beneficial bacteria as a side effect.

The hospital-acquired C.diff colitis infection is an example of an antibiotic-induced imbalance of bacterial flora, in which the patient experiences repeated bouts of painful and severe diarrhea due to overgrowth of the Clostridium difficile bacteria following the use of a broad-spectrum antibiotic to treat a different condition. C. diff. is life-threatening if not treated successfully.

A more common and less severe example is vaginal yeast infections following the use of antibiotics for throat or urinary tract infections.

Other medications such oral contraceptives produce a change in our intestinal pH, which leads to an abundance of certain bacterial strains and scarcity of others.

Stress

Researchers have also found that stressful conditions can increase the number of pathogenic bacteria present in the gut. Stressful situations cause a release of the neurochemicals epinephrine (Epi) and norepinephrine (NE), our fight or flight chemicals, also known as adrenaline and noradrenaline, respectively, which can spill into the intestines.

Stressful situations that trigger NE such as anger and fear lead to increased growth of E.coli, Yersinia Enterocolitica and Pseudomonas aeruginosa. Additionally, under stressful conditions, E. coli releases a substance that is essentially a "growth hormone" for other Gram-negative bacterial species, letting other potentially pathogenic bacteria know that it is their time to "multiply and attack.[6]"

These stressful situations create a favorable environment for the often pathogenic Gram-negative bacteria, and one that is less favorable to the survival of the beneficial bacteria such as the Lactobacillus species.

Numerous studies and case reports have found that exacerbation of intestinal disorders tends to occur after a stressful period, and we now understand that the types of bacteria that reproduce during stressful times may be responsible for the symptoms.

Diet

Changes in diet, even small ones, can have an impact on the type of bacteria that thrive. A 15-gram-a-day diet addition of oligofructose or inulin (fructose-based dietary fibers) lead to the bacteria Bifidobacterium to be found as the predominant bacterial species in the feces of individuals studied. Prior to the addition of inulin, Bacteroides, Clostridia, and Fusobacteria were the predominant species present.

According to Elaine Gotschall, the author of "Breaking the Vicious Cycle," a diet rich in refined carbohydrates can lead to a compromised GI flora. Anecdotal evidence has shown that people who become affected with intestinal disorders were more likely to eat a diet high in simple carbohydrates compared with those who were not affected.

What Happens When the Normal Flora Becomes Imbalanced?

In this shift toward the proliferation of unfriendly bacterial species, the excessive fermentation byproducts that these bacteria produce lead to damage of the intestinal tract, damaging the delicate microvilli containing the brush border enzymes that are responsible for digestion. According to Elaine Gotschall, the intestinal walls may produce more mucous as a protective mechanism from the damage. The excess mucous then coats the brush border enzymes and forms a barrier between the food and the enzymes inhibiting digestion.

In other cases it has been reported that the mucous border may diminish, exposing the intestinal wall to damage. When bacteria become imbalanced, the overgrowth of pathogenic bacteria will lead to damage of the endothelial lining, as pathogenic bacteria produce their own enzymes that break down the protective mucous coat of the intestinal lining as well as degrade the pancreatic and brush border enzymes.

The first enzyme that becomes affected is the enzyme lactase (which is used to break down the lactose sugar found in milk). It is also the last enzyme to regenerate once the bacterial world is stabilized. Interestingly, statistics claim that 70% of people are deficient in this enzyme, which leads this author to wonder whether lactose-intolerant people are also suffering from a gut microflora imbalance.

While certain carbohydrates such as monosaccharaides (single sugars) can be absorbed by the body to provide nutrition without needing to be digested, disaccharides (double sugars) and polysaccharides (multiple sugars), cannot be digested or absorbed without the activity of brush border enzymes, which cleave them into the absorbable monosaccharide components.

These undigested carbohydrates remain in the intestinal tract and are utilized as "lunch" for the bacterial universe. The pathogenic bacteria ferment the carbohydrates and this leads to flatulence, gas, and bloating and further intestinal damage, creating the "vicious cycle" described by Elaine Gottschall.

Furthermore, without proper digestion and the aid of beneficial bacteria, the person may become malnourished or have vitamin/mineral deficiencies despite adequate intake.

B_{12} deficiency may result from this malabsorption, which further contributes to the "vicious cycle," as B_{12} is required for the growth and proper function of villi. Other nutrients that are important to thyroid health, such as selenium, zinc and omega-3 fatty acids may also become depleted.

TESTING

Stool tests are available to check microbial balance. The tests can tell us whether there is a lack of beneficial bacteria or an overabundance of pathogenic organisms such as potentially pathogenic Gram-negative species or Candida.

These same tests can be used to check for Yersinia Enterocolitica.

I recommend the GI Effects Profile from Metametrix, which also tests for digestion/absorption, gut immunology, metabolic parameters, parasites as well as the mixture of intestinal flora. This test helps to determine microbial balance by quantifying the amounts of beneficial and pathogenic bacteria.

You may also add on the Full GI Panel option when ordering parasite tests from Parasitetesting.com which will show potentially pathogenic bacteria in addition to parasites. This test is very comprehensive for a variety of pathogens and Yersinia is always included in this panel. However, the limitation of this test is that beneficial bacteria are not shown.

The tests can be very helpful in determining your course of action. For example, I found that although I had plenty of Bifidobacteria, I had zero Lactobacilli! I also had an overgrowth of E. coli and Proteus Vulgaris, which have both been implicated in autoimmunity.

SMALL-INTESTINAL BACTERIAL OVERGROWTH

Small Intestine

The small intestine has millions of tiny mucosal fingerlike projections called villi that line the intestinal wall. These villi are made from epithelial cells and are covered with the even smaller microvilli that make up the brush border cells "the fuzzy fringe." These cells contain brush border enzymes that digest carbohydrates, proteins, and fats (amylase, lactase, maltase, and sucrose are some examples). The space between the epithelial cells is called a tight junction. Under normal conditions, food is transported into the small intestine where it is further worked on by brush border enzymes.

Figure 9: The Intestinal Tract

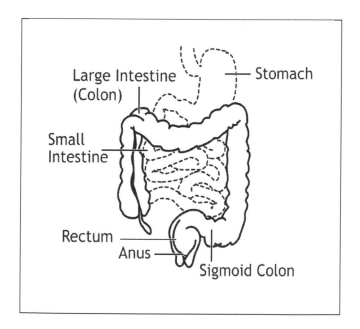

Diagram of the Human Intestine. Drawn by Duncan Lock and released into the Public Domain. Available at http://commons.wikimedia.org/wiki/File:Intestine-diagram.svg Accessed March 29, 2013

Large Intestine

The large intestine is also known as the colon. Resident bacteria of the colon depend on the host to feed them, especially with carbohydrates that were not digested/absorbed in the small intestine, such as starches, polysaccharides, fiber, sugars, and oligosaccharides. The colon bacteria ferment undigested foods, mucous, sloughed epithelial cells, and pancreatic enzymes for energy to help themselves grow and multiply.

Bacteria from the colon may also creep up into the small intestine where they can cause an overgrowth. Small intestinal bacterial overgrowth (SIBO) has been associated with a variety of gastrointestinal conditions such as Crohn's disease and IBS. It is also a potential cause of increased intestinal permeability.

Generally, the small intestine is supposed to have fewer bacteria than the colon, but in some cases (following food poisoning, for example) more bacteria may get into the small intestine. Hydrogen breath tests are available to test for overgrowth of bacteria in the small intestine.

FOOD AND INTESTINAL PERMEABILITY

When one has a leaky gut the food is never properly digested. Instead, food particles can also cross the intestinal barrier and get into the circulation. Just like the bacteria, these substances in our circulation become recognized as "invaders" by our immune system, and the immune system launches a white blood cell (WBC) attack, leading to the development of food intolerances that can be measured as IgG antibodies to these foods, similar to the antibodies formed to the endotoxins produced by bacteria.

Somehow, either the bacteria or the foods are cross-linked with thyroid peroxidase (bystander effect) and the immune system begins to develop IgG antibodies to TPO. As time goes on, the foods and bacteria act as environmental triggers that perpetuate the IgG antibodies. (More about this in the "Intolerance" chapter).

The Gluten Autoimmune Connection

Certain proteins may induce an immune system response. The most well-described is the gluten intolerance seen in celiac disease. Gluten is a protein found in wheat that causes intestinal damage and thus destroys the intestine's ability to absorb nutrients in people with gluten intolerance. What researchers are now finding is that gluten intolerance may be a spectrum, with many people being intolerant but not testing positive when receiving the screening tests.

The other issue with some of the screening tests is that they measure your body's intestinal IgA response to gluten. In some advanced cases, your intestines may be so damaged that the IgA will be too depleted to create an immune response. In that case, the person will test negative for gluten intolerance. If a biopsy was done of the intestines (which is a much more expensive and invasive procedure that would not likely be done unless there was a positive screen result), it would show that the intestines were severely damaged.

The best test for gluten intolerance, or any other intolerance, is removing it from your diet for a few weeks followed by a challenge when you reintroduce the suspected food.

If you have Hashimoto's, you likely have some degree of gluten intolerance and need to remove gluten from your diet. Some people may have the same type of reaction to casein and whey in dairy products. Others may have this type of reaction to the protein found in eggs or soy.

I know that I personally tested borderline for gluten intolerance, but positive for dairy protein intolerance. I felt much better after taking both out of my diet, and this change was an essential part of my recovery. A re-challenge with both foods did indeed confirm my sensitivity.

Although celiac disease is five to fifteen times more common in people with Hashimoto's compared with the general population, non-celiac gluten intolerance is also a factor in many autoimmune conditions. Gluten also has a direct on intestinal permeability, even in the absence of celiac disease.

Symptom improvement in many autoimmune conditions has been reported after the initiation of a gluten-free diet. Length of gluten exposure is positively associated with the development of autoimmune conditions. This means that the longer you eat gluten, the more likely you are to develop an autoimmune condition! Some researchers have found that three to six months on a gluten-free diet can eliminate organ-specific antibodies, such as those to the thyroid seen in Hashimoto's. Some individuals have reported that their TPO antibodies disappeared after getting rid of gluten, without any other lifestyle changes. Thus, a three to six month gluten-free trial should be undertaken by everyone with an autoimmune condition.

When Did the "Staff of Life" Become So Toxic?

The rates of celiac disease, autoimmune conditions, and gluten intolerance are increasing in many countries including the U.S. and Europe.

Traditional bread preparation techniques involved using a "sourdough" fermentation process that would break down the gluten protein. This process involves putting a special type of yeast on the flour that takes about three days until the bread is ready to be baked.

Conventional bread preparation techniques don't bother with this process and most wheat products in breads, cereals, and processed foods contain gluten.

Small studies have shown that breads prepared from wheat in a traditional sourdough process appeared to be safe for people with celiac disease. Additionally, another study showed that these types of beneficial bacteria produced in the fermentation of breads might actually promote healing for those with celiac disease [42-46].

So what is celiac disease, gluten sensitivity, and how does it relate to Hashimoto's?

Celiac disease is an autoimmune condition, where eating gluten, a protein found in wheat, barley, and rye causes the body to attack the lining of the small intestine.

The attack on the intestines destroys the villi, which are delicate hair-like projections that cover the intestines and help to digest and absorb nutrients from food.

This damage of the villi causes the person with celiac/gluten intolerance to become malnourished, no matter how much food he or she eats, because the body is not able to absorb the nutrients from the food that is consumed. Villi also contain enzymes that help us digest food, so celiac disease could impair the digestion of many other foods, especially those containing lactose.

HEALING INTESTINAL PERMEABILITY

In order to heal autoimmune conditions, we need to reduce intestinal permeability. This is achieved through removing offending agents and rebalancing depletions that are preventing our bodies from working optimally. We must also take away the habits and stressors that cause depletions.

Taking antibiotics to target the Gram-negative bacteria may be helpful in some cases, but may not always solve the root cause of the problem and may also further compromise the bacterial balance in our intestines.

Dr. Maes has found that in combination with a leaky gut diet, antioxidants like glutamine, n-acetyl cysteine, and zinc can help "tighten" the intestinal tight junctions within one year.

Additional antioxidants were also utilized: L-carnitine, coenzyme Q10, taurine, lipoic acid, (in case of carnitine and/or coenzyme Q10 deficiency), gamma oryzanol, curcumin, and quercetin (in the case of systemic or intracellular inflammation) as well as a "leaky gut diet" that was described as gluten-free, dairy-free, and low-carb.

According to Dr. Maes, "natural anti-inflammatory and anti-oxidative substances may improve the integrity of the gut barriers by reducing gut-derived inflammation and tightening the opened tight junction barrier."

Glutamine

Glutamine is the best-studied substance for healing intestinal permeability. A deficiency in glutamine is also known to cause increased intestinal permeability in mouse models and malnourished children.

Glutamine supplementation has been found to reduce the damage and leaky gut associated with the use of NSAIDS, and has been found to reduce gut permeability in patients who underwent abdominal surgery.

New epithelium in the GI is produced in three to six days, and glutamine can help repair the GI lining and works together with other amino acids, such as leucine and arginine. Glutamine needs to be taken orally to be effective.

Glutamine dosed at 0.5 grams/kg ideal body weight per day for two months was shown to reduce intestinal permeability in subjects with Crohn's disease. Dr. Maes used a more conservative dose of 7 grams per day.

Zinc

Zinc supplementation has also been shown to tighten leaky gut in other conditions such as Crohn's disease. Maes, et. al., found that zinc levels were lower in those with chronic fatigue syndrome. Other studies showed that zinc can be lowered by the presence of increased level of pro-inflammatory cytokines such as IL-6. Furthermore, low zinc has been associated with hypothyroidism. The dose used by Dr. Maes was 30 mg per day.

N-Acetylcysteine (NAC)

Glutathione is an antioxidant that is deficient in those with Hashimoto's. It helps prevent free radical damage to the thyroid, but isn't well absorbed if taken orally. N-Acetylcysteine (NAC) is a precursor to glutathione, and can be taken orally. NAC has been used for healing intestinal permeability, however, it can cause stomach upset if taken on an empty stomach and thus should be taken with food. Dr. Maes used a dose of 1.8 grams per day with chronic fatigue patients.

Factors that reduce intestinal permeability

- Beneficial bacterial species from probiotics and fermented foods
- N-Acetylcysteine
- AT-1001 (Larazotide)
- Black pepper, green pepper, nutmeg, bay leaf (peperine)
- Black tea
- Protamine
- Glutamine
- Zinc
- Quercetin
- Saturated fat
- Medium chain fatty acids
- Lauric acid and palmitic acid
- Butyrate
- Leaky gut diet

Rebalancing the Bacterial Flora

Most people with Hashimoto's have imbalanced bacterial flora. This seems to be the root cause of many autoimmune conditions contributing to intestinal permeability and increased autoimmunity. Thus the strategy to overcome autoimmune conditions is to rebalance the bacterial flora, which will lead to a normalization of intestinal permeability. When our bacterial flora is not balanced, this contributes to the autoimmune condition through continuous antigen stimulation.

Rebalancing the bacterial flora can be done through medications, diets, and probiotic and digestive enzyme supplementation.

Diets (Refer to the Diet Chapter for more information).

1) A two-week elemental diet, where an easily digestible liquid formula is consumed in place of food has been shown to reduce small-intestinal bacterial overgrowth. However, the liquid diet may be a drawback for those with high blood glucose or those who are underweight.
2) The specific carbohydrate diet and GAPS diet are diets that limit the consumption of fermentable carbohydrates, which will slowly rebalance the flora.
3) Daily consumption of lacto-fermented foods such as sauerkraut and kimchee, which contain beneficial bacteria, will, over time, displace the pathogenic bacteria.

Probiotics

Probiotics are used to rebalance the normal flora. Just as with fermented foods, the beneficial bacteria in probiotics should help displace the pathogenic bacteria.

When starting probiotics and fermented foods, it is recommended to start small and gradually increase the dosage until a die-off reaction is felt.

A die-off reaction, also known as a Jarisch-Herxheimer reaction, or sometimes just Herxheimer or "Herx," is a reaction that occurs when in their death, the pathogenic bacteria release endotoxins at a quicker rate than the body can clear them (read more about bacterial toxins in the "Alkaline Phosphatase" chapter).

If die-off is too severe, the dose may be reduced a bit, but generally it should resolve within three to five days, while the probiotic dose is continued.

Symptoms of die-off may include: lethargy, difficulty concentrating, craving sweets, diarrhea, rash, irritability, gas, bloating, headache, nausea, vomiting, congestion and increased autoimmune symptoms.

The dose of probiotic may need to be reduced if the die-off is severe, to prevent more autoimmune damage, or immune modulation may be attempted to desensitize the body from the toxic effects. (See the "Immune Imbalance" chapter).

When choosing a probiotic, the following are important considerations:

1) Multiple strains of beneficial bacteria (not just L. acidophillus)
2) Concentration of active bacteria expressed as CFUs (colony forming units). These should be in the billion range per capsule.

Examples of Beneficial Bacteria Species (Probiotics)	
Bacillus subtilis	Lactobacillus delbrueckii
Bifidobacterium bifidum	Lactobacillus DDS-1
Bifidobacterium breve	Lactobacillus helveticus
Bifidobacterium infantis	Lactobacillus lactis
Bifidobacterium longum	Lactobacillus plantarum
Lactobacillus acidophilus	Lactobacillus reuteri
Lactobacillus brevis	Lactobacillus rhamnosus
Lactobacillus bulgaricus	Lactobacillus salivarius
Lactobacillus casei	Streptococcus thermophilus

The downside of diet, probiotics, and supplements is that they take six months to two years to change the bacterial flora. In the meantime, the autoimmune process may still be propagating. Thyroid medications, elemental diet, and immune modulation (see Chapter 15) are crutches we can use to help us along the way during our healing journey.

Pre-Biotics

Fiber is poorly digested by all humans, and usually serves as food for our gut bacteria. You may have heard about pre-biotic fibers like inulin and FructoOligoSaccharide (FOS) that are used alongside probiotics to feed the good bacteria and encourage them to grow. Unfortunately, in the presence of gut dysbiosis, this wonderful food gets eaten by the bad guys instead. This is why I do not recommend prebiotics in the case of dysbiosis. Additionally, while fiber is a healthy component of a balanced diet, in some cases, fiber may need to be restricted altogether for a period of time in order to heal dysbiosis. Diets such as the FODMAPs or Low Residue Diet that limit fiber are further discussed in the Diet Chapter.

Saccharomyces boulardii

Levels of IgA can be increased by taking the beneficial yeast Saccharomyces boulardii which helps clean up the intestines. S. boulardii does not take up residence in the intestines, but does a lot of great work passing though.

Digestive Enzymes

Pathogenic bacteria feed on foods that we do not digest properly. This is especially an issue with sulfate-reducing bacteria that ferment protein to form a toxic gas that damages our intestinal lining. As most people with Hashimoto's are low in hydrochloric acid, leading to poor protein metabolism, adding in a digestive enzyme will help us break down foods properly. This way we get the nutrients from the food we eat and starve the pathogenic bacteria.

Medications

Antibiotics-According to Dr. Allison Siebecker, who has created a website dedicated to sharing information about small-intestinal bacterial overgrowth (www.siboinfo.com), the antibiotics Metronidazole, Rifaximin (Xifaxan™), and Neomycin have been used to treat small-intestinal bacterial overgrowth because of their ability to stay in the intestines, which prevents them from causing systemic adverse events.

Larazotide- While alternative medicine has been suggesting a link between leaky gut and autoimmune conditions for years, traditional medicine finally started to take notice after the discovery of zonulin, a potential drug target.

By modifying the interaction between gene expression and environmental triggers through re-establishing the intestinal barrier function, the autoimmune processes can be arrested. This is supported in both animal models and recent clinical trials, and provides a new approach to treat and prevent autoimmune diseases.

AT-1001 (Larazotide), a zonulin blocker, has shown promise in preventing reactions to gluten in patients with celiac disease—this type of drug has great marketing potential as its effect on blocking zonulin will likely be temporary, leading the patient to require the drug on an ongoing basis. If larazotide is an effective zonulin blocker, it will likely become the next blockbuster drug generating billions of dollars in profits for the pharmaceutical industry through chronic disease management of autoimmune conditions. At the time of writing this book, Larazotide was available in limited clinical trials for refractory celiac disease, and preliminary results were positive.

Luckily, we don't have to wait until this drug gets FDA approval, as there are already permanent lifestyle approaches that can heal intestinal permeability in many cases.

Perfect Storm for Type 1 Diabetes

Type 1 Diabetes, also known as Insulin Dependent Diabetes Mellitus (IDDM), is analogous to Hashimoto's. Both conditions start with circulating autoantibodies. In IDDM, the antibodies are to the beta cells in the pancreas, while in Hashimoto's the antibodies are to thyroid peroxidase (TPO).

Over time these antibodies start destroying their target and leading to a loss of production of the necessary hormone, insulin in the case of IDDM, and thyroid hormone in the case of Hashimoto's.

Lymphocytic infiltration of the target organ occurs in both autoimmune conditions, where white blood cells accumulate in the beta cells and thyroid tissue in IDDM and Hashimoto's, respectively.

In the case of IDDM, increased intestinal permeability has been identified to be present before the onset of beta cell destruction.

A trio of factors has been suggested to form the "Perfect Storm" in Type 1 Diabetes pathogenesis: abnormal microbial flora, leaky intestinal mucosal barrier, and an altered immune system in intestinal cells.

The role of microbiota has been established in the Type 1 diabetes (but not Type 2 diabetes) disease model as well. Certain types of bacteria have been associated with autoimmune disease incidence, while other types of bacteria were protective of it.

Interestingly, when fecal matter from mice whose flora protected them from diabetes was transplanted into mice who previously had not had the protective bacteria in their guts, they too were less likely to develop diabetes.

Recently, dairy and gluten consumption has been implicated in the development of Type 1 diabetes. Studies were done when hydrolyzed casein, (a type of rapidly absorbing partially digested milk protein that bypasses the stomach and is absorbed by the small intestine) was given instead of cow's milk to children who were genetically susceptible to develop IDDM. These children were less likely to develop IDDM by 40%, compared with children who were fed cow's milk.

Additionally, children with diabetes were found to have intestinal immune activation, and not just the children with the HLA DQ2 gene that is associated with celiac disease.

Elimination of gluten did not eliminate the intestinal immune activation, although immune reaction was found when exposed to gluten and dairy. This leads us to believe that intestinal permeability leads to an altered response to food and microflora-derived antigens. In other words, the increased intestinal permeability comes first, followed by an altered response to foods.

My Story

I first became gluten free after having learned about normalization of TPO antibodies in some people after eliminating gluten. However, I was not one of those lucky people. Although I felt much better, I continued to have elevated TPO antibodies despite complete avoidance of gluten, dairy, and soy for almost two years.

I was able to eliminate Candida after about six months of a Candida diet. What really helped was actually cutting out fruit and taking biotin 5,000 mcg, which keeps Candida in its non-infectious form. Biotin becomes depleted in adrenal insufficiency and causes hair loss, so it was one supplement that worked overtime for me and achieved a triple score. But that did not eliminate my antibodies, either.

So I dug deeper. I ordered additional tests and found out that I had dysbiosis with an overgrowth of Proteus Vulgaris. I learned that Proteus species bacteria are implicated in autoimmunity as well as what they like to eat: fructose and undigested meat. I had been following a leaky gut diet for about a year, but did not see improvement until I made some tweaks that were specific to my situation. I cut out fruit, added digestive enzymes and fermented cabbage and began to experience severe die-off symptoms within a couple of days, which signaled the beginning of my healing crisis!

Chapter Summary

✓ Increased intestinal permeability must be present to develop an autoimmune condition.

✓ The bacterial universe in our guts controls the immune system.

✓ Bacterial overgrowth/imbalance, gluten, alcohol, food intolerances and other factors cause intestinal permeability.

✓ Removing gluten from the diet is recommended for everyone with an autoimmune condition.

✓ Pathogenic bacteria can damage our intestinal lining.

✓ Leaky gut diet, medications, supplements, probiotics, and fermented foods can be helpful in restoring bacterial balance and intestinal permeability.

✓ Rebalancing the bacterial makeup through diet and introduction of more Gram-positive bacteria may help reduce inflammation and autoimmunity.

"The best and most efficient pharmacy is within your own system." -Robert C. Peale

12: ALKALINE PHOSPHATASE

In the previous chapter, we learned that the commensal bacteria in our bodies create toxins and may be implicated in autoimmunity. Alkaline phosphatase deficiency is another piece of the puzzle that results in autoimmunity.

What is Endotoxin?

Endotoxin is also known as lipopolysaccharide (LPS) and is a component of the cell walls of Gram-negative bacteria. Gram-negative bacteria are present in varied amounts in the intestines of animals and humans, with variability between 7% and 50% of the total bacterial species.[5] These bacteria can either be pathogenic and cause serious illnesses, or may live in balance with our normal flora and may be considered "opportunistic." Opportunistic bacteria behave well when they are surrounded by Gram-positive beneficial bacteria, but may become naughty when they don't have the Gram-positive bacteria to keep them in line.

Endotoxin from Gram-negative bacteria can promote inflammation through the stimulation of Th-1 pro-inflammatory cytokines (TNFa) in the intestine, as well as the rest of the body, especially in those with intestinal permeability. LPS in the circulation can cause inflammation and even septic shock if present in great amounts.

Pro-inflammatory cytokines are seen with many autoimmune conditions, including Hashimoto's, Type 1 diabetes, inflammatory bowel disease, and celiac disease. Endotoxin is thus being considered a promoter of autoimmune conditions.

Alkaline phosphatase

Alkaline phosphatase (AP) is an enzyme found in our bodies that works to take away phosphate groups from a variety of molecules. One of the roles of AP is to detoxify LPS from Gram-negative bacteria. AP removes phosphorous from the cell wall of the bacteria and thus detoxifies the endotoxin. AP enzymes are anti-inflammatory and have evolved to help us tolerate our resident microbes by making us less reactive to them.

Crohn's disease and colitis are thought to be caused by an abnormal immune response to Gram-negative resident bacteria in the intestine. Antibiotics effective for Gram-negative bacteria are utilized for treatment of these conditions, and these conditions have also been associated with reduced levels of alkaline phosphatase. Researchers have found that giving rats oral alkaline phosphatase enzymes showed a reduction of inflammation.

Having enough alkaline phosphatase helps us to prevent an immune response to our gut bacteria. When we are low in alkaline phosphatase, our body is not able to detoxify the bacteria present in our ecosystem, and thus we may have inflammatory reactions.

LAB TESTING

Standard liver function panels will include a test for alkaline phosphatase. If you have had a liver function panel, you have likely had your alkaline phosphatase measured.

Elevated levels of alkaline phosphatase may be found in cases of infection, liver damage, or other serious conditions. In contrast, low levels of AP are rare in general practice, so your physician may not have known what to do with them. I know I was told not to worry about my low alkaline phosphatase levels by multiple physicians, as only high levels of alkaline phosphatase were relevant to them. Thus, had I not seen my own lab results, I would have never searched for an answer and made this connection.

Low alkaline phosphatase levels are usually associated with malnutrition (nutrient deficiencies), and are commonly found with hypothyroidism and Hashimoto's. Thyroid hormones induce the production of more alkaline phosphatase.

Intestinal damage due to gluten and other intolerances, low stomach acid, and other conditions commonly present in Hashimoto's put people at risk for malnutrition because of poor protein assimilation.

For example, studies found that people with untreated celiac disease, and thus a high degree of intestinal damage that affects their ability to absorb nutrients from food, have reduced AP activity in the intestinal mucosa compared with people with normal intestinal function. Alkaline phosphatase activity correlated with the degree of damage, meaning, that this one test could show just how damaged the intestines were. In people with Celiac disease, the enzyme activity began to normalize after the initiation of a gluten-free diet and once the intestinal lining began to heal and absorb nutrients again.

Nutrient deficiencies associated with low alkaline phosphatase include: vitamin B_6, B_{12}, folic acid, vitamin C, phosphorous (usually a genetic condition detected at birth), zinc, and protein.

Fasting, fat-free diets, low-protein diets and unsaturated fats also reduced AP. The inclusion of saturated fats, short chain fatty acids (butyrate), and medium chain triglycerides (coconut oil) increased AP.

The amino acids L-cysteine and L-phenylalanine (found in artificial sweeteners) are potent inhibitors of AP. Additionally, phytates found in legumes and grains reduce AP enzyme activity as does guar gum, a common food additive.

Excessive soda consumption may be associated with reducing AP levels. Sodas also have very high phosphatase amounts and are known for leaching calcium from our bones. Studies done on chicks found that low dietary phosphorous increased the activity of AP by 50%, compared with adequate phosphorous levels.

In contrast, fermented foods and the Gram-positive probiotics such as Lactobacillus casei stimulate alkaline phosphatase' as do saturated fats, fiber and carbohydrates alkaline phosphatase activity. [6]

Smoking, which has been found to be protective of developing Hashimoto's, increases alkaline phosphatase. [7]

Various blood types may be associated with AP levels. Individuals with Type O blood seem to secrete the most, while those with Type A blood, the least. [8]

Alkaline phosphatase works best in a more alkaline (or basic) environment with a pH in the range of 9–10. Note: While the stomach should be acidic, the rest of the body should to be slightly alkaline for optimal body function. [4]

Increasing Alkaline Phosphatase Activity

Restoring depletions is required for increasing low alkaline phosphatase. People with Hashimoto's, even if overweight, are usually experiencing nutrient deficiencies because they are not extracting nutrients from their foods correctly.

Increasing the right foods is the first obvious step, but it is also imperative to make sure that we are absorbing nutrients from our food correctly.

If your alkaline phosphatase is low, you likely have gluten or another type of intolerance that is causing inflammation in your intestines. Additionally, you are likely not digesting proteins correctly and potentially have low stomach acid.

Reducing the amount of Gram-negative bacteria may also be helpful with relieving inflammation. Thus, taking a probiotic supplement and fermented foods rich in Gram-positive bacteria will help establish a better balance. Taking Gram-positive probiotics will decrease Gram-negative bacteria that secrete LPS.

Short chain fatty acids such as butyrate, derived from butter or from fermentation of dietary fiber in the gut may also be helpful for increasing AP.

Nutrient Dense Foods to Include in Your Diet
- Saturated Fats: animal fats, coconut oil
- Zinc: oysters, pumpkin seeds, ginger root, pecans, peas, Brazil nuts
- B_{12}: protein (make sure you are digesting correctly)
- Vitamin A: liver, carrots, pumpkin, salmon oil, cod liver oil
- Fish oils: omega-3, -6, and -9, either as a supplement or from fresh seafood such as herring, salmon, sardines, and cod liver oil
- Vitamin A: carrots, sweet potatoes, pumpkins
- Butyrate: butter, dietary fiber (forms butyrate on fermentation in gut)
- Alkalizing foods: fresh fruits and veggies
- Increase Gram-positive bacteria: lacto-fermented foods, drinks, and probiotics)

Minimize AP inhibitors

Potential ways to minimize AP inhibitors are a grain-free/legume-free diet such as the Paleo, GAPS, or SCD Diet, or soaking and cooking grains and legumes to reduce phytates as recommended in the Body Ecology Diet.

Reducing the intake of soda and diet sodas that contain artificial sweeteners and phosphorous as well as reducing processed foods is also recommended.

Create an Alkaline Environment in the Body

As alkaline phosphatase works best in an alkaline body environment, increasing alkalizing foods may help with making the enzyme more efficient. Green juices are a great and delicious way to alkalize. They are absorbed well and do not feed the pathogenic bacteria. Just about everyone can tolerate them. (More about juicing and alkalizing foods in the "Toxins" chapter).

Chapter Summary

- ✓ Endotoxin is a toxic substance produced by Gram-negative bacteria that live in our intestines
- ✓ Alkaline phosphatase is an enzyme that detoxifies endotoxins.
- ✓ People with hypothyroidism usually have low alkaline phosphatase.
- ✓ Increasing alkaline phosphatase may be helpful in neutralizing endotoxins from Gram-negative bacteria.

"The part can never be well unless the whole is well". -Plato

13: ADRENALS

Hypothalamic Pituitary Adrenal Axis and Hashimoto's

The hypothalamus is our command center for hormones. It sends messages to the pituitary to control various organs such as the liver, thyroid, adrenals, mammary glands, and ovaries. This is why adrenal fatigue and hypothyroidism often go hand in hand.

The hypothalamic-pituitary-adrenal (HPA) axis is an intricate system of direct and indirect feedback mechanisms that regulate the body's reaction to stress. The HPA axis also plays a major role in regulating the immune system, digestion, energy usage, mood, and sexuality. The HPA is controlled by hormones, which are altered when the body experiences stress.

Treating hypothyroidism without treating a dysfunctional HPA Axis is one of the biggest reasons people continue to feel exhausted despite receiving treatment with thyroid hormones. Patients may initially report feeling more energetic, but this is usually followed by feeling worse and worse until they are right back to where they were before they started the thyroid medications. They will go back to their physicians to check blood work and will be told that everything is normal.

The patient begins to feel crazy ... but that's when another layer of what is broken in Hashimoto's becomes unraveled. Many symptoms of hypothyroidism actually overlap with symptoms of underactive adrenals, however, physicians don't routinely check adrenal function in those with Hashimoto's.

Symptoms of poor adrenal function may include the following:

feeling overwhelmed, feeling tired despite adequate sleep, difficulty getting up in the morning on most days, craving for salty foods (a.k.a. "I just ate a whole bag of chips syndrome"), increased effort required for everyday activities, low blood pressure, feeling faint when getting up quickly, mental fog, alternating diarrhea/constipation, low blood sugar, decreased sex drive, decreased ability to handle stress, slowed healing, mild depression, less enjoyment in life, feeling worse after skipping meals, increased PMS, poor concentration, reduced ability to make decisions, reduced productivity, poor memory ... do any of these sound familiar?

The Adrenals

The adrenal glands are almond-sized organs that sit on top of each kidney. Each gland has two separate zones. The inner zone, or medulla, secretes the hormones epinephrine (Epi), also known as Adrenaline; Norepinephrine (NE), and a small amount of dopamine in response to immediate stress signaled by the central nervous system.

The outer zone of the adrenal gland is known as the cortex. The cortex secretes three types of hormones; glucocorticoids, mineralocorticoids and androgens. These hormones are made from cholesterol, are essential to everyday life and are secreted in varied amounts throughout the day.

Glucocorticoids

Cortisol is the main glucocorticoid and is stimulated by the release of adrenocorticotropin hormone (ACTH) from the pituitary gland. The primary functions of cortisol are to help regulate blood sugar levels, increase body fat, defend the body against infections, and help the body adapt to stress. Cortisol also helps to convert food into energy and has anti-inflammatory properties.

Mineralocorticoids

Aldosterone is the main mineralocorticoid. It helps with regulating blood volume, blood pressure, and the body's sodium and potassium levels.

Androgens

Dehydroepiandrosterone (DHEA) and testosterone are androgen hormones present in both men and women. Women produce DHEA and testosterone in both the adrenals and the ovaries.

DHEA has been touted as the "youth" hormone, as its production peaks around age 20 and decreases over time. By age 40 our bodies make about half the amount of DHEA as they used to, by age 65, 10%-20%, and by age 80 that drops to less than 5% of the amount produced at age 20. DHEA increases production of insulin-like growth factor 1 (IGF-1), which is a signal for human growth hormone, a powerful anti-aging hormone. DHEA enhances the body's ability to fight off infections and higher levels have been associated with reduced self-antigens. DHEA protects the body from the effects of cortisol and the stress that triggers its production.

The adrenal glands are responsible for manufacturing hormones from cholesterol. These types of hormones are also known as steroids. Cholesterol becomes converted into pregnenolone. Pregnenolone is the precursor for DHEA, estrogen, testosterone, progesterone, aldosterone, and cortisol.

The adrenal cortex secretes varied amounts of hormones throughout the day in a rhythmic pattern, with the highest amounts in the morning, and the lowest at night. When the adrenal glands are not putting out sufficient amounts of hormones or the rhythm becomes disturbed, adrenal dysfunction develops.

Figure 10: Steroid Hormone Synthesis

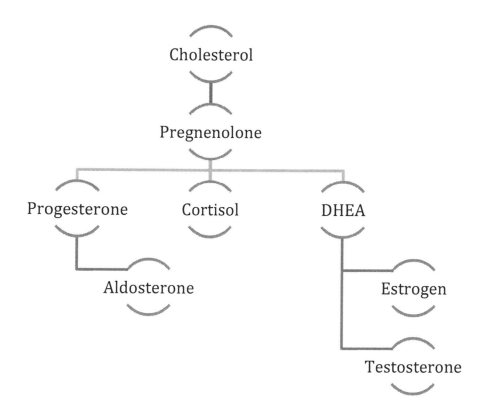

Stress and Adrenal Function

Stress is linked to most chronic illnesses. We already discussed what happens to the bacterial universe when we are feeling angry, fearful, or sad. However, stress affects other parts of our body as well, contributing to the development of autoimmune diseases.

Under normal conditions, our body creates an adaptive stress response via the HPA Axis and the sympathetic nervous system (SNS). Let's explore what happens to the HPA axis when we are stressed.

Immediate Stress Response

The hypothalamus is our stress sensor in the brain. Once stress is perceived, the hypothalamus will set off a hormone cascade that leads to the activation of our fight or flight response (via the sympathetic nervous system). The adrenals are our stress response glands, and release stress hormones.

Chronic Stress

During stressful situations, the body will shift hormone production away from the progesterone/aldosterone pathway, and away from the DHEA/estrogen/testosterone pathway to focus on producing cortisol. This mechanism is known as "pregnenolone steal," where the body will take the pregnenolone that is normally reserved for DHEA and progesterone and put it towards cortisol production. This is a protective way of conserving resources to help us survive stressful fight or flight situations like car crashes, being chased by bears, and the like.

This "reserve fuel function" is a brilliant design or evolution of the human body and is extremely important in times when we are fighting or running for our lives. However, a near-death experience is not always necessary to turn on the fight or flight response, and it can turn on in situations we find stressful in modern times that are not necessarily life-threatening, like running late, being stuck in traffic, or having to give a presentation at work. This can then turn into a chronic activation of the stress response.

Your body will work extra hard to keep producing more cortisol, and even stop the production of other hormones that are normally produced by the adrenals such as progesterone, DHEA, and testosterone. The precursor for all of these hormones and cortisol is pregnenolone. Your body will start "stealing" the pregnenolone that would normally be reserved for progesterone and DHEA production to keep up the supply of cortisol.

Chronic stress leads to three distinct stages of adrenal fatigue. In the initial stage, the HPA will be over-responsive, and is known as the High Cortisol Stage. At this time the total cortisol will be high, and the DHEA will be borderline, low, or normal. Left unchanged, this stage can progress into the second stage, the Cortisol Dominant State, where DHEA will be either low or borderline, and the cortisol will be normal. As this continues, eventually the adrenals become exhausted and start to burn out, progressing to the third stage, the Low Cortisol Stage. In this stage the DHEA will be either low or borderline low, and the total cortisol will be low.

Putting hormone production on hold for prolonged periods of time can be quite problematic.

In beginning stages of chronic stress, blood pressure may be normal if the body adequately compensates, or it may become elevated if the body is not able to rebalance the hormonal response. In the advanced stages of adrenal fatigue, aldosterone production becomes depleted and levels of sodium and water drop, resulting in low blood pressure. The person may also feel faint upon standing.

Figure 11: Stress Response Cascade

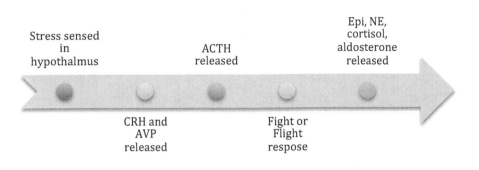

1) The hypothalamus senses stress and releases the corticotropin releasing hormone (CRH) and arginine vasopressin (AVP) hormones.
2) These hormones trigger the production of adrenocorticotropic hormone (ACTH), which activates the fight or flight response.
3) This triggers the release of norepinephrine and epinephrine from the adrenal medulla, and signals the adrenal cortex to produce cortisol and aldosterone.
4) Epinephrine constricts our blood vessels and increases blood pressure to make sure our brain is receiving enough blood and oxygen to deal with the "impending danger."
5) Cortisol acts as an anti-inflammatory hormone, preventing damage from the inflammation of other substances that are released during stress and has the important job of maintaining and preserving fuel to keep us going in the case of a crisis that requires energy, by increasing levels of glucose through stimulating production of new glucose from the liver and causing insulin resistance. Insulin resistance helps us keep more glucose around, and therefore keeps us fueled up with energy.
6) The main task of aldosterone is to regulate how much fluid is stored in our bodies. Fluid volume in turn also has an effect on blood pressure. The more aldosterone we have, the more sodium and water we retain, and thus aldosterone helps with keeping the blood pressure up.

People may become dehydrated and will start craving salty foods (hello potato chips). The level of potassium may actually become relatively higher, causing an imbalance, thus foods containing high potassium may make the person feel worse. Simply drinking more fluids will result in further dilution of the sodium and further dehydration.

Chronic stress leads to a reduction in DHEA and progesterone. These hormones are often abnormally low in individuals suffering from autoimmune diseases like inflammatory bowel disease and rheumatoid arthritis, as well as CFS and fibromyalgia. Additionally, seasonal depression, post traumatic stress disorder, hypothyroidism, asthma, and eczema have all been linked to HPA axis malfunction.

Low progesterone can lead to menstrual irregularities, infertility, uterine fibroids, fibrocystic breasts, as well as a shift in immune function. Progesterone regulates GABA, our "relaxation hormone", and a deficiency in GABA can lead to anxiety, insomnia, and rumination (rumination means excessive worry about the past).

DHEA has been touted as an anti-aging hormone, and has been correlated with reversing the classic stress-induced physiological response. In stressful situations, to make enough cortisol ACTH will drive elevated levels and deplete DHEA production to adapt. Without enough DHEA, the body won't be able to produce enough testosterone, which can affect the sex drive.

While DHEA levels drop with age, various diseases including autoimmune conditions, cancers, diabetes, heart disease, dementia, and chronic fatigue have been associated with low DHEA. When DHEA levels are down, our immune system becomes more sensitive to pathogens and free radicals.

When secreted in excess, cortisol injures the body's tissues. The main role of cortisol is to keep the body fueled up during a stressful time. Cortisol will shift the body into a tissue breakdown phase (catabolic), instead of a tissue repair phase (anabolic). In normal conditions this should be balanced. DHEA is an anabolic steroid and helps with tissue repair, counterbalancing the effects of cortisol. However, DHEA becomes depleted during the chronic stress response.

Chronic cortisol release can result in the depletion of many nutrients that affect our physiology. Cortisol releases amino acids from the muscles to help create more glucose. One of these amino acids is glutamine, which is very important for the maintenance of the gut lining integrity and has been found to be depleted in people who have leaky gut. Additionally, excessive cortisol output causes a reduction in Secretory IgA (SIgA). SIgA is secreted in various mucosal surfaces and helps with viral and toxin neutralization and stopping bacterial colonization in the gut. Thus, excess cortisol makes it more likely for us to pick up a gut infection.

Cortisol also inhibits vitamin D activity, preventing calcium absorption. This leads to the breakdown, instead of building, of bones. Cortisol also leads to impaired detoxification due to inhibition of liver function.

Additionally, prolonged cortisol can cause many issues, including more secretion of pro-inflammatory cytokines, poor wound healing, easy bruising, infertility, central obesity, and mood and memory disorders due to increased turnover of neurotransmitters.

When cortisol runs out and the rest of the body is depleted, a sickness response occurs; fatigue, impaired cognition, sleep disturbances, anorexia, and depressed mood can occur. As cortisol has anti-inflammatory and immune suppressive effects, the person may become more susceptible to allergies and inflammation.

Low cortisol results in a lack of suppression of sympathetic tone and catecholamines, thus we are more sensitive to the effects of epinephrine and may experience anxiety, an increased sense of smell, and a heart rate that is elevated, or on the higher end of normal (this should be noted as a symptom of HPA dysfunction in people with Hashimoto's, as hypothyroidism is associated with a slower heart rate).

The level of cortisol controls thyroid hormone production. Often low thyroid symptoms such as fatigue and low body temperature are due to an adrenal maladaptation.

What is Stress?

There are **four** types of stress that turn on our fight or flight response; mental/emotional stress, sleep disorders, metabolic/glycemic dysregulation, and chronic inflammation.

Mental Stress

Feelings such as grief, guilt, fear, anxiety, excitement, and embarrassment can be classified as stress. This stress is based on our perception, not on the nature of the individual stress. For example, public speaking may cause plenty of mental stress for someone with social anxiety, but another person who enjoys speaking in front of others may perceive the experience as pleasurable. Situations that are new, unpredictable, threaten the ego, or when a loss of control is felt, are perceived as stressful.

Glycemic Burden

Researchers in Poland have found that up to 50% of patients with Hashimoto's have an impaired tolerance to carbohydrates. This means that after consuming carbohydrate-rich foods, their blood sugar levels would spike up very high, causing a great amount of insulin release. The role of insulin is to clear blood sugar out of our cells, so a large insulin release is followed by a rapid drop of blood sugar (hypoglycemia). Symptoms of hypoglycemia are very unpleasant and may include irritability, fainting, lightheadedness, or tremors. Hypoglycemia necessitates the release of cortisol to help maintain the glucose supply to the brain and counteracts insulin, causing insulin resistance (this is also linked to the Type 2 diabetes epidemic).

Sleep Disorders

Sleep deprivation is used in lab animals to suppress the HPA Axis. Sleep deprivation can be caused by insomnia, sleep apnea, and shift work. Enough said. Sleep is the reset button for the HPA Axis. When we sleep, our body releases human growth hormone and repairs itself. Make sure to get at least seven hours of sleep each night and be tested for sleep apnea if you snore.

Inflammation

Chronic inflammation may occur from joint pain, obesity, toxic burden, inflammation in the GI tract, from irritable bowel disorders, pathogens in the GI tract, or food allergies. These conditions will signal cortisol for its anti-inflammatory effect.

HPA Dysfunction and Autoimmunity

Some researchers believe that HPA axis dysfunction and prolonged cortisol elevation may be the *cause, rather than the consequence* of autoimmune diseases. Cortisol is a natural steroid and suppresses cellular immunity (Th-1), preventing tissue damage from excessive inflammation.

Low cortisol allows for up-regulation of cellular immunity (Th-1 dominance), resulting in the increased production of pro-inflammatory cytokines TNF-A, IL-6, IL-12. During Th-1 dominance, the Th-2 branch (humoral immunity) is suppressed. This may lead to the person becoming more susceptible to parasites, allergens, bacteria, and toxins. Th-1 dominance is often seen in autoimmune conditions.

Thus, the immune system may become thrown out of balance in times of excess cortisol production and when cortisol is depleted. Pregnant women's cortisol was measured at week thirty-six of gestation. Those with low cortisol levels were more likely to develop postpartum thyroiditis.

Thus stress, along with nutritional deficiencies and intestinal permeability, may be at the root cause of Hashimoto's and may perpetuate the disease progression.

TESTING FOR ADRENAL FATIGUE

Adrenal Quiz (Adapted from Adrenal Recovery Kit)

1 point for each yes

☐ Do you frequently have low body temperatures? (<98 degrees F)
☐ Do you frequently get irritable?
☐ Do you have poor memory or concentration?
☐ Do you notice palpitations?
☐ Do you suffer from allergies or asthma?
☐ Do you bruise easily or find your wounds heal slowly?
☐ Do you get frequent/chronic infections?
☐ Do you have dry, thinning skin?

Continued on next page…

- [ ] Do you get headaches?
- [ ] Do you have unexplained hair loss?
- [ ] Do you skip meals?
- [ ] Do you exercise more than one time each week?
- [ ] Do you have thyroid problems?
- [ ] Is your energy good all day?
- [ ] Do you need caffeine in the morning or after lunch?

3 points for each yes

- [ ] Are you emotionally overstressed?
- [ ] Do you get tenderness across your lower back?
- [ ] Do you suffer from depression or down moods?
- [ ] Do you have low blood pressure?
- [ ] Do you experience a "second wind" (high energy) at bedtime?
- [ ] Do you experience chronic or recurrent inflammation?
- [ ] Do you get light headed when sitting up or standing?

5 points for each yes*
(*yes to any of these should trigger an adrenal test)

- [ ] Do you suffer from chronic pain?
- [ ] Do you suffer from low blood sugar/hypoglycemia? (i.e., headaches, sleepiness, mood swings if skipping meals)
- [ ] Do you suffer from insomnia?
- [ ] Do you experience symptoms of PMS? (breast tenderness, abdominal cramping, heavy periods, mood swings)
- [ ] Are you menopausal or peri menopausal? (skipped periods, between 45 and 55 years old, hot flashes, vaginal dryness)

If your score >10 you probably have some degree of adrenal dysfunction

If your score >20 it is highly probably you have adrenal dysfunction

If your score >30 it is nearly certain you have adrenal dysfunction

Blood pressure test

People with adrenal fatigue often have low blood pressure and/or a drop in blood pressure after standing up from a lying down or sitting position (orthostatic hypotension).

If your blood pressure is below 120/80 mmHg, this may mean that your adrenals are underactive, or that you are dehydrated.

Orthostatic hypotension test: While lying down or siting, relax and deep breathe for at least five minutes, and then measure your blood pressure, then stand up and measure again. Normally, you should see a rise in blood pressure. If you see a drop in blood pressure, you may be dehydrated or have underactive adrenals. Symptoms may include dizziness or lightheadedness when standing up from a sitting/lying down position.

Pupil Contraction

People with low adrenal function may often have difficulty with contracting their pupils. Usually our pupils dilate (enlarge) in the dark, and contract (get smaller) in the light.

You can try the following test with a flashlight: Stand in your bathroom with the lights out for a few minutes, allowing your eyes to adjust. Shine the flashlight across your eye, keeping the flashlight perpendicular to your face (do not shine the light directly into your eyes) and watch how your pupils react.

Normally, the pupils should get smaller and stay that way. If they get smaller then bounce back and forth only to become slightly bigger again, this may be a sign of poor adrenal function. Symptoms may include light sensitivity, difficulty seeing in bright lights, and having to wear sunglasses.

Unstable Temperatures

If you are keeping track of your basal temperatures, low and unstable morning temperatures may be suggestive of adrenal insufficiency.

Hormone Testing

Adrenal hormones can be measured through blood or saliva testing. Saliva testing, which measures the "free" or available hormones of cortisol throughout the day as well as levels of DHEA, progesterone and estrogen, is often used to detect adrenal fatigue. Blood tests may also be utilized to test for hormone deficiencies, however, blood tests may not always detect adrenal fatigue, as they do not pick up changes until 90% of the adrenal cortex has been destroyed.

Thyroid Function and the Adrenals

Cortisol inhibits the peripheral conversion of T4 to T3, the active thyroid hormone. At the same time, it promotes the production of reverse T3 (rT3), an inactive thyroid molecule that still has three iodine molecules, but in the *wrong* spaces (see Figure 12).

This molecule is able to bind the receptor sites that T3 normally occupies, but it does not have the ability to *unlock* these receptors, thus not allowing the necessary reactions to take place.

At the same time, cortisol prevents the release of TSH, preventing the production of more thyroid hormones. Thus, when we take a lab test, we will see that our TSH may be "normal," and even the T3, T4 may be normal, but we will still be having thyroid symptoms.

Most physicians don't test for reverse T3, but this test is readily available and can be easily added to a thyroid blood panel test.

Figure 12: T3 and Reverse T3 Molecules

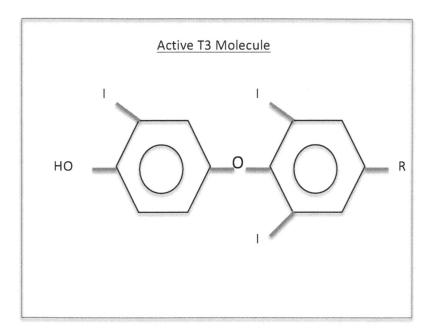

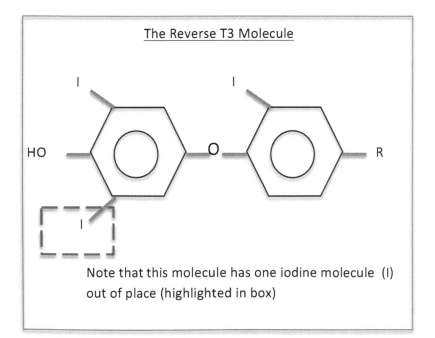

Thyroid Supplements

Once thyroid activity increases (as a result of thyroid supplements or lifestyle interventions) there is additional stress put on the adrenals, resulting in worsening of symptoms. This can make most people feel like they are suffering a huge setback despite making gains-thus addressing adrenals should always be considered in conjunction with restoring nutritional deficiencies when attempting to improve thyroid function.

Addison's Disease

Full-blown adrenal insufficiency is also known as Addison's disease, and is usually not diagnosed until someone is going through an adrenal crisis (an emergency situation). Addison's disease used to be historically associated with tuberculosis and other types of infections that destroyed the adrenal glands. Today, autoimmunity is the leading cause of Addison's, responsible for 70%-90% of cases, with corresponding anti-adrenal antibodies. The most common antibody is formed to one of the adrenal enzymes, 21-hydroxylase, and up to 86% of patients with autoimmune adrenal insufficiency will be positive for these antibodies.

Symptoms of full-blown Addison's include weakness, fatigue, loss of appetite, weight loss, darkening of the skin, nausea, vomiting, low blood pressure with orthostatic hypotension (dizziness when standing), muscle and joint pain, salt cravings, decreased hair growth in underarms and pubic area, and diminished sex drive in women. These symptoms are similar to those of adrenal fatigue, but are more severe is most cases, sometimes requiring hospitalization. Physicians screen for adrenal fatigue by checking to see if there is an elevation of ACTH or by measuring blood levels of cortisol or DHEA. Adrenal insufficiency becomes clinically manifest only after at least 90% of the adrenal cortex has been destroyed.

Subclinical Addison's

People with Hashimoto's and other autoimmune conditions are more likely to develop Addison's.

Co-occurring Addison's and Hashimoto's is known as Schmidt's disease, and any person with Hashimoto's who has anti-adrenal antibodies should be considered to have both conditions.

People with anti-adrenal antibodies will go on to develop adrenal insufficiency at a rate of 19% per year. Some people with the antibodies were followed for more than thirty-five years and never developed the full-blown adrenal insufficiency. The concentration of autoantibodies correlates strongly with the degree of adrenal dysfunction. However, most physicians don't typically screen patients with Hashimoto's for anti-adrenal antibodies. So your adrenals could be breaking down right before your eyes and you might not even know about it...

Addison's is not usually diagnosed until a significant amount of the adrenal glands has been destroyed by autoimmune damage, however, many Hashimoto's patients actually present with symptoms of adrenal insufficiency, which are often mistaken for symptoms of hypothyroidism.

While conventional medicine does not recognize "adrenal fatigue" as a diagnosis, I would like to propose that perhaps some of the individuals with Hashimoto's who have symptoms of adrenal fatigue actually have subclinical Addison's, where the adrenals are in the process of being destroyed, but the hormonal changes may not be significant enough to be detected on blood tests or the body may still be compensating.

Just like TSH is a measure of thyroid activity, ACTH elevation signals adrenal distress. Cortisol is the active hormone of the adrenals, just as is free T3 of the thyroid. However, one can have a normal TSH, normal free T3 and still have hypothyroid symptoms, and thus we would recommend a TPO antibody test. Just the same, it may be helpful to request a 21-hydroxylase autoantibody test despite normal ACTH levels and normal blood cortisol levels.

It is not clear if the cause of adrenal insufficiency or Subclinical Addison's is due to depletion, down regulation, or autoimmune origin, however, adrenal function and thyroid function have an impact on one another.

TREATMENT OF HPA DYSFUNCTION

Recovery from HPA dysfunction may take three months to two years. Treatment goals should focus on correcting the deficiencies that were caused by excessive cortisol production and removing HPA stressors. The use of adaptogens and glandular extracts may be helpful. In some cases, hormonal or pharmacological treatment may need to be used.

- Correcting deficiencies: cholesterol, co-factors, B vitamins, salt
- Supplementing the hormone production: adaptogens, glandulars, hormones
- Removal of stressors: this step is the hardest but the most important.

ADRENAL DEPLETIONS

Dehydration

As many people with adrenal fatigue may have suboptimal sodium retention and hydration due to aldosterone levels being low, people may become dehydrated and will start craving salty foods (such as potato chips). The level of potassium may actually become higher, thus foods containing high potassium may make the person feel worse. Simply drinking more fluids will result in further dilution of the sodium.

Liberal use of non-iodized sea salt is recommended, and drinking filtered water with one teaspoon of non-iodized sea salt may be helpful. Homemade chicken broths with plenty of sea salt are also a great and tasty way to rehydrate.

Cholesterol

Adrenal hormones are made from cholesterol. Adequate cholesterol is important to have in your diet. Egg yolks and meat are the richest sources of dietary cholesterol that can be eaten by people with autoimmune thyroid conditions.

Nutrient Depletion

Vitamin C and B vitamins become depleted during high cortisol production. Pantothenic acid and biotin deficiency in particular have been linked to decreased adrenal function in animals and humans. Potassium, zinc, iron, and copper also become depleted with excessive cortisol production.

People with adrenal dysfunction may be deficient in the following:
- Vitamin C
- Niacin
- Pantothenic acid
- Folic acid
- Biotin
- Potassium
- Zinc
- Iron
- Copper
- Magnesium

While some may wish to obtain these supplements from natural whole-food sources, due to gut issues people with Hashimoto's usually have an impaired ability to extract vitamins and minerals from food. It may be helpful to take a supplement in the beginning, until gut function is restored.

Supplements are not created equally, and many multivitamin tablets have questionable absorption profiles. I don't like recommending "One a Day"-type vitamins because they don't consider how the vitamins interact with one another. For example vitamin C taken together with iron improves the absorption of iron, while iron taken together with zinc decreases the absorption of zinc. Thus providing just the RDA of zinc when only 50% of it will be absorbed will not be effective in overcoming a severe zinc deficiency. Some vitamins/minerals may also need to be taken with food to promote absorption, others on an empty stomach.

SUPPORTING HORMONE PRODUCTION

Adaptogenic Herbs

Adaptogenic herbs can be any natural herb products that supplement the body's ability to deal with stressors. In the 1940s Dr. Nikolai Lazarev defined adaptogen as "an agent that raises the body's ability to resist stress by countering undesired stressors, whether physical, chemical, emotional, or biological."

Most adaptogens have been used for thousands of years in Eastern medical practices, such as Ayurveda and traditional Chinese medicine (TCM).

A variety of herbs can be used as adaptogens, and can be formulated by herbalists for specific patients based on the symptoms.

In order to be considered an adaptogen, an herb must possess several qualities.

First, the herb must be nontoxic to the patient at normal doses.

Second, the herb should help the entire body to cope with stress.

Third, the herb should help the body to return to "normal" regardless of how stress is currently affecting the person's functioning.

In other words, an adaptogen herb needs to be able to both tone down overactive systems *and* boost underactive systems in the body. Adaptogens are thought to normalize the hypothalamic-pituitary-adrenal (HPA) axis.

Adaptogenic herbs include ashwagandha, astragalus reishi mushroom, dang shen, eleuthero, ginseng, jiaogulan, licorice, maca, schizandra, spikenard, and suma. These are examples of herbs that may increase the body's ability to resist stress, and have been helpful in relieving adrenal dysfunction when used in combination with vitamins and minerals.

Licorice root extract prevents the breakdown of cortisol into inactive cortisone. Thus, keeping cortisol around longer will prevent the body from stealing pregnenolone from production of other hormones and may be helpful for adrenal insufficiency. It also may be beneficial for those with low cortisol and low blood pressure. It should not be used by those with water retention or high blood pressure.

Adrenal supporting supplements will usually have a mix of the various herbs, and some may also contain vitamins and/or glandular extracts.

Adaptogenic Herbs
American ginseng (*Panax quinquefolius*)
Amla (*Emblica officinalis*)
Ashwagandha (*Withania somnifera*)
Asian ginseng (*Panax ginseng*)
Astragalus (*Astragalus membranaceus*)
Chaga mushroom (*Inonotus obliquus*)
Cordyceps (*Cordyceps sinensis*)
Dang Shen (*Codonopsis pilosula*)
Guduchi (*Tinospora cordifolia*)
He Shou Wu (*Polygonum multiflorum*)
Holy basil (*Ocimum sanctum*)
Jiaogulan (*Gynostemma pentaphyllum*)
Licorice (*Glycyrrhiza glabra*)
Lycium (*Lycium chinense*)
Maca (*Lepidium meyenii*)
Prince Seng (*Pseudostellaria heterophylla*)
Reishi (*Ganoderma lucidum*)
Rhaponticum (*Rhaponticum carthamoides* or *Stemmacantha carthamoides*)
Rhodiola (*Rhodiola rosea*)
Schisandra (*Schisandra chinensis*)
Scutellaria baicalensis
Shatavari (*Asparagus racemosus*)
Shilajit (*Asphaltum bitumen*)
Siberian Ginseng (*Eleutherococcus senticosus*)
Suma (*Pfaffia paniculata*)

Supplemental Hormones:

Based on the results of the cortisol saliva test and the stage of adrenal insufficiency, a variety of hormones and adrenal supporting substances may be utilized. Although most of these hormones are available over the counter at health food stores, they are certainly not benign and should be used under the supervision of a trained professional with **extreme caution**. Not everyone will need all of these supplements.

One person may do fine only with glandular extracts, another may need to add DHEA, another person may not need any of these hormonal supplements at all. It is very individual. It is especially important to start low and go slowly with these supplements. People should start one supplement at a time at the lowest dose, and increase every few days to get to the target dose. After the first supplement has been tolerated for a week, another one may be added. The doses provided here are for reference purposes and may not be appropriate for all persons and stages.

Many hormones, including cortisol and thyroid hormone, are controlled by a feedback loop system that shuts off production when levels get high. Not so with DHEA and pregnenolone: Your body will keep right on making these hormones in the same amounts as before you began supplementation. In other words, taking supplements of DHEA and pregnenolone won't suppress your body's production of these hormones or cause adrenal atrophy.

Glandular Adrenal Extracts

Adrenal extracts have been used medicinally since 1931. Similar to Armour thyroid (which is derived from pig thyroid glands), pig, sheep or cow adrenal glands are made into adrenal extracts in tablet and capsule form for human ingestion. Commercially available adrenal extracts are made from the whole gland (whole or total adrenal extracts) or just from the outer part of the gland (adrenal cortex extracts). Adrenal extracts are usually taken one to three times per day.

These extracts are not FDA-regulated and not all are created equally. The whole-gland adrenal extracts contain norepinephrine and epinephrine, which can cause anxiety, palpitations, and panic attacks in Hashimoto's patients who may already have too much epinephrine without enough cortisol to balance it out. Adrenal cortex extracts may be preferred for those who are already feeling on edge.

Adrenal extracts can cause HPA axis suppression and atrophy. Meaning, they can turn off the production of the body's own steroid (adrenal) hormones, and potentially thyroid hormones by pituitary feedback loop inhibition. Thus, the pituitary may stop sending out messages to the adrenals and thyroid to produce more hormones. This may result in central hypothyroidism, which is an abnormally low TSH (in the levels of hyperthyroidism), coupled with low levels of both free T3 and T4. The person who initially feels better with adrenal glandular extract only to crash a few weeks to months later with symptoms of hypothyroidism and a "normal" or "low" TSH should be suspected of HPA axis suppression. In this case, the adrenal glandulars need to be tapered down slowly, at about 10%-20% reduction in dose every four days to one week. Rapid withdrawal may cause symptoms like pain, low blood pressure, extreme fatigue, nausea, and a rebound effect of the thyroid condition.

HPA suppression is more likely to happen at prolonged doses that are higher than the normal physiological output of adrenal hormones normally produced, and especially if dosed at bedtime. As the pituitary usually releases TSH to stimulate thyroid production at night, adrenal extracts should never be taken at bedtime.

Remember, even though they are natural, glandulars are still steroids and should be taken only under the supervision of a trained health-care professional.

Pregnenolone

Pregnenolone is the precursor to many of the hormones produced by the adrenal cortex, and often gets "stolen" in order to produce more cortisol. Pregnenolone supplements may be given to those who are low in progesterone, aldosterone, or DHEA. They should be used with extreme caution in those with elevated and normal levels of aldosterone or who are currently experiencing any fluid retention, swelling, or bloating. Unlike some of the other hormones, aldosterone production doesn't turn off when there is too much of it, so pregnenolone may lead to aldosterone excess, which can cause fluid retention and extremity pain due to nerve compression. Any signs of fluid retention or pain warrant stopping the supplement. The fluid retention should resolve after the pregnenolone is stopped. The pain may persist for many weeks, requiring adequate rest and rehabilitation.

Progesterone

If the results of hormone tests show low progesterone, and if the woman is experiencing cycle irregularities, infertility, or other types of concerns, progesterone supplements may be utilized. Again, as excess progesterone may turn into aldosterone, the same precautions pertaining to fluid retention should be exercised.

DHEA

DHEA supplementation increases stress tolerance, lowers the cortisol/DHEA ratio, and protects against cortisol-induced cellular damage. DHEA supplementation has been found to extend the lifespan of animals, and has shown much promise in various conditions, including adrenal insufficiency.

Unlike pregnenolone, DHEA does not turn into aldosterone so it wouldn't cause fluid retention, however, it may be converted to testosterone.

DHEA stimulates hair follicles and oil glands, so it may cause acne, or facial hair growth in women. (Teenage acne has recently been connected to a rise in DHEA that takes place near puberty).

Additionally, some people may become more irritable and theoretically may become more aggressive due to the testosterone conversion. These side effects should go away with dose reduction or discontinuation.

7-Keto is an active metabolite of DHEA that is not able to convert into testosterone, so some professionals prefer to use the 7-Keto version of DHEA to minimize side effects.

Yam extracts containing diosgenin are touted as natural sources of DHEA, however, the DHEA is not bioavailable to humans, thus we can't convert the diosgenin from the yams to active DHEA in our bodies.

DHEA levels should be tested prior to supplementing. Testing is covered by most insurance companies if ordered by a physician.

The recommended daily dose range is 10–50 mg for women, 25–100 mg for men. (Women need less DHEA than men.) However, starting low and slowly increasing should always be the approach. Some professionals give women even less DHEA, as low as 2 5mg/day.

DHEA should be supplemented until the levels reach those of a 30-

year-old of the same gender: (200 and 300 micrograms per deciliter of blood for women) and (300 and 400 micrograms per deciliter of blood for men).

Topical Magnesium Therapy

According to Dr. Norm Shelley, M.D., PhD., using topical magnesium oil can be used to increase DHEA levels in as few as four to five weeks without having to take an oral DHEA supplement. Many of us are deficient in magnesium, and oral supplementation is not always a reliable way to increase levels. Using magnesium may not be appropriate for those with impaired kidney function, but may be a more natural way to increase the body's DHEA production. The magnesium oil is not technically an oil but a solution. Using 2–4 oz. in a bath or a twenty- to thirty-minute foot soak is recommended to restore intracellular magnesium levels. Epson salt baths have also been found to increase magnesium levels.

Conventional Treatment for Addison's Disease

Addison's disease is diagnosed by measuring morning levels of cortisol via a blood test. If the cortisol level is low, this confirms Addison's. Conventional treatment for Addison's is supplementing with hormones, including prescription steroid hormones like prednisone, cortisone, and hydrocortisone. The over-the-counter supplement DHEA also may be used in Addison's.

Blood tests for Addison's will not be positive until 90% of the adrenals are destroyed, and thus some people may have 70% of their adrenal cortex destroyed but still come out "normal" on cortisol blood tests.

Some physicians may prescribe the prescription steroid hormones used in Addison's for people with adrenal insufficiency.

REMOVING STRESSORS

"Give me the strength to change what I can, the patience to accept what I cannot, and the wisdom to know the difference."- Reinhold Niebuhr

We have all heard that "stress is bad for your health," but it has often been one of those vague generic statements that people never take to heart.

Stress can be emotional such as being in an unstable romantic relationship, being a high-strung person with high expectations of yourself and others, being overbooked, multitasking, or having a job you don't enjoy. Stress can also be physical, such as working long hours, extreme sports, not getting enough sleep ...

Removing stressors does not require the purchase of any special supplements or medications, but may be the most difficult step for most people. Most of us are not at liberty to quit our stressful jobs, send our teenagers away to boarding school, or purchase an airplane to forgo traffic. But we can choose how the stressors affect us. After all, it is our *perception,* not the stressors themselves that determine how the HPA reacts to them.

Above all, stress is about perception. What do you perceive as stressful in your life? Write down a list of things that you find stressful, and whether these stressors are things you should or could get rid of, or if you need to re-evaluate your approach to how you perceive these stressors.

Try to avoid these: pushing yourself past the point of being tired, caffeine, sugar, alcohol, flour, staying up past 11 p.m., being hard on yourself, feeling sorry for yourself ...

Some strategies to reduce stress include...

1. Read self-help books on relaxation, overcoming stress, etc. "How To Stop Worrying And Start Living" by Dale Carnegie is a great classic.
2. Find one thing to be thankful for each day.
3. Listen to books on CD while doing things you don't enjoy. For example I despise traffic and cleaning the house. Listening to a book on CD keeps my busy mind engaged instead of worrying about the traffic or the house.
4. Music: Try the Spa station on Pandora for instant relaxation!
5. Meditation, yoga, and tai chi are all relaxing hobbies.
6. Cut out toxic people ...
7. Get organized and simplify your life.
8. Consume less: turn off the TV, get off the Internet, stay out of stores.
9. Take time for yourself ... daily, weekly, monthly, yearly.
   a. Daily: Try a yoga class, hot bath, or closing your eyes for 15 minutes to meditate.
   b. Weekly: Schedule a day off from work—a day when you just do what you want to do. You are forbidden from running errands, doing chores, or work. Do you feel like reading all day? Do it! Do you want to stay in bed all day? Do it! Do you want to get a mani-pedi? Go for it. It's your time, your body, your health. One strategy for those of us who are lucky enough to have time off from work is to "schedule" your sick days. Schedule work responsibilities around the planned sick day.
   c. Monthly: Schedule a message/spa day with the girls.
   d. Yearly: Schedule a beach vacation, schedule a staycation!
10. Control freaks ... learn to let it go. You can't rest the weight of the world on your shoulders. Retire from your position as CEO of the Universe. You will be much better off and surprisingly, the world will go on.

11. Mindfulness: Pausing, and being present and observant of how things are affecting you can be a great way to learn how to relax yourself.
12. Avoid getting overtired and/or overexcited
13. Laugh several times a day.
14. Enjoy life, get a pet.
15. Do your best to eliminate, simplify, delegate, automate.
16. Be more resilient by being more flexible. Bruce Lee said "Notice that the stiffest tree is most easily cracked, while the bamboo or willow survives by bending with the wind."
17. Do the things that you like.
18. Orderliness and predictability are your friends. Plan your life that way when you can. Catch up on bills, checkbooks, and your long to-do lists. Keep your space neat and clean. Schedule times to clean the house and catch up on life, not just big events. Make sure you schedule down time as well.
19. Avoid burning the candle at both ends.
20. Massage, acupuncture may help get you relaxed.
21. Avoid multitasking. Do one thing at a time and keep your full attention on it before you move on to the next task. Take a small break in between tasks.
22. Start a journal, make your own list, be mindful of what makes you feel better, what makes you feel worse.

My plan. Daily: do relaxing activity like taking a hot bath, going on a long walk, listening to relaxing music, meditating, yoga class (see the chapter on Finding Your Root Cause on creating your own list).

Adequate Rest

Sleep is regenerative and crucial to adrenal recovery. It is important to go to sleep by 10 every night and sleep for at least eight hours. Sleeping until 8 or 9 a.m. whenever possible may also be helpful to the recovery process. A good bedside hygiene should be practiced. A room that is completely dark with all electronic devices switched off will maximize melatonin production. The use of stimulants such as coffee, caffeinated beverages, and even TV and the computer may need to be limited.

Artificial light, such that comes from television and computers may trick our retinas into thinking that it is light outside, thus halting the production of melatonin, a hormone that promotes restful sleep. Shutting off televisions/computers three hours before going to sleep is recommended.

People who wake up in the middle of the night and are unable to sleep may benefit from a small dose of melatonin or magnesium at bedtime.

Exercise

Mild to moderate exercise is helpful for adrenal insufficiency. Exercise helps calm the mind, reduces stress, and increases blood flow, leading to better oxygenation and detoxification throughout the body and helping to normalize levels of hormones. Additionally, exercise can help stabilize blood sugar imbalances and people may find that they are less likely to have blood sugar spikes when eating carbohydrates right after exercise.

For those who are currently sedentary, setting a goal of walking for 20 minutes once a week or going to one yoga class per week would be a great start, gradually increasing to three times per week.

Extreme exercise, such as training for a marathon or triathlon, may be too demanding for someone who is undergoing adrenal fatigue, and may need to be postponed until after the person recovers.

Stimulants

Coffee, alcohol, and tea (except for herbal tea) may need to be avoided. Caffeine stimulates ACTH, which in turn stimulates the adrenals and cortisol production.

Blood Sugar Imbalances

Balancing blood sugar levels should be one of the priorities for anyone who is hoping to overcome autoimmune thyroiditis and adrenal fatigue.

Insulin is released to lower our blood sugar levels. We have learned that many people with Hashimoto's have an impaired tolerance to carbohydrates. Their blood sugar goes up too high, too quickly after eating carbohydrates. This leads to a rapid, sometimes excessive release of insulin. These insulin surges can cause low blood sugar (reactive hypoglycemia), which can cause unpleasant symptoms such as nervousness, lightheadedness, anxiety, and fatigue.

Reactive hypoglycemia is a stressor for the adrenals.

Cortisol is released when the adrenals become stressed, and excess release of cortisol can also produce an immune imbalance. When this pattern of excessively high and then low blood sugars keeps happening, we may also develop insulin resistance. Insulin resistance leads to Type 2 diabetes, another American epidemic.

What Puts us at Risk for Having a Blood Sugar Imbalance?

Unfortunately the Standard American Diet (SAD) is perfectly designed to produce an epidemic of diabetics, as well as people with autoimmune conditions.

Having a fast-paced lifestyle that leads to skipping breakfast, having "liquid" lunches, consuming a high-carbohydrate, low-fat diet, and of course the excessive sugar consumption is the norm. It's not our fault. Unfortunately, there's is a lack of education on the topic of nutritious eating. This essential should be taught right along with history, math, and English from an early age. Instead, Americans rely on commercials and marketing to tell them what is healthy and what is not. For example, Subway subs, Yoplait yogurt, and Gatorade are marketed as healthy and nutritious even though they are full of sugar!

During pharmacy school we learned about nutrient requirements in our first year Biochemistry course. I was shocked to learn that carbohydrates were not a required nutrient, while fat was required for normal cell function! Based on my previous nutrition knowledge gathered from store displays, the USDA Food Pyramid and Subway commercials I was led to believe that carbohydrates were the most important and fats needed to be avoided.

I am sure I was not the only person misled by the "low fat" labeling of foods and the prominent placement of carbohydrates as the base of the Food Pyramid. Fortunately, the new USDA MyPlate no longer encourages people to eat the equivalent of one loaf of bread on a daily basis. However, we still have a long way to go.

This is evident by the number of people seen with diabetes, obesity and chronic disease in the United States. Our fat-phobic society has been on a fat-free craze, without the realization that excess fat does not turn into fat, it turns into a rather unpleasant case of diarrhea, while excess carbohydrates are stored as fat!

Every system is perfectly designed to get the results it gets. Thus, our current society is designed to produce an epidemic of people suffering from diabetes, obesity and chronic diseases. Perhaps we need to redefine our recommendations to produce better results.

What is the Glycemic Index?

The glycemic index is a measure of how quickly food becomes assimilated into our bodies. You can also call it the "burn" rate, how quickly we burn the fuel we receive from these foods.

Carbohydrates have a very quick burn rate. They become assimilated very quickly into our bodies, which causes a rapid and high spike in blood sugar. After eating carbohydrates we become hungry again after less than an hour.

Fat and protein have a slower burn rate. They become assimilated into our bodies more slowly and gradually and don't raise blood sugar levels as quickly. They also keep us full longer. Assuming enough calories eaten to feel full, a person will be hungry again two to three hours after eating protein, and four hours after eating fat.

Figure 13: Blood Sugar Elevation Following Consumption of High GI or Low GI Foods

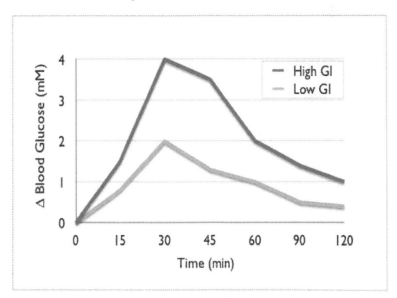

Do You Have a Blood Sugar Imbalance?

Symptoms of Blood Sugar Imbalance
(adapted from "The UltraMind Solution")

- ☐ I crave sweets and eat them, and though I get a temporary boost of energy and mood, I later crash.
- ☐ I have a family history of diabetes, hypoglycemia, or alcoholism.
- ☐ I get irritable, anxious, tired, and jittery, or get headaches intermittently throughout the day, but feel better temporarily after meals.
- ☐ I feel shaky two to three hours after a meal.
- ☐ I eat a low-fat diet but can't seem to lose weight.
- ☐ If I miss a meal, I feel cranky and irritable, weak, or tired.
- ☐ If I eat a carbohydrate breakfast (muffin, bagel, cereal, pancakes, etc.), I can't seem to control my eating for the rest of the day.
- ☐ Once I start eating sweets or carbohydrates, I can't seem to stop.
- ☐ If I eat fish or meat and vegetables, I feel good, but seem to get sleepy or feel "drugged" after eating a meal full of pasta, bread, potatoes, and dessert.
- ☐ I go for the breadbasket at restaurants.
- ☐ I get heart palpitations after eating sweets.
- ☐ I seem salt sensitive (I tend to retain water).
- ☐ I get panic attacks in the afternoon if I skip breakfast.
- ☐ I am often moody, impatient, or anxious.
- ☐ My memory and concentration are poor.
- ☐ Eating makes me calm.
- ☐ I get tired a few hours after eating.
- ☐ I get night sweats.
- ☐ I am tired most of the time.
- ☐ I have extra weight around the middle (waist to hip ratio > 0.8; measure around the belly button and around the bony prominence at the front of the top of the hip).

Continued on next page....

- [ ] My hair thins in the places I don't want it to (my head) and it grows in the places it shouldn't (my face, if I am a woman).
- [ ] I have a family history of polycystic ovarian syndrome or am infertile.
- [ ] I have a family history of high blood pressure.
- [ ] I have a family history of heart disease.
- [ ] I have a family history of Type 2 diabetes (what used to be known as adult-onset diabetes).
- [ ] I have chronic fungal infections (jock itch, vaginal yeast infections, dry scaly patches on my skin).

Achieving Blood Sugar Balance

While the treatment of advanced cases of glucose metabolism dysregulation such as diabetes is beyond the scope of this book, healthy eating that promotes a stable blood sugar is a necessary component of preventing and treating diabetes and hypothyroidism.

Eating a low glycemic index diet helps with feeling fuller longer, improves cholesterol levels, blood sugar levels, improves cognitive performance, improves energy, and reduces acne. It also reduces your risk of developing diabetes, heart disease, some cancers, and promotes weight loss for those who are overweight. Many people have also found their moods improve after balancing their blood sugar.

The following quick reference chart can make balancing your blood sugar much easier.

Type of Food	Until you are hungry again
Protein	2-3 hours
Fat	4 hours
Carbohydrate	45 minutes-1 hour

Glycemic Index

The glycemic index of foods can be referenced at www.glycemicindex.com. Foods with a glycemic index of less than 55 are considered to have a low glycemic index and include most non-starchy vegetables, meats, nuts, seeds, and some whole grains. The fruit with less fructose—"sour" fruit such as grapefruit, lemons, limes and cranberries also have a low glycemic index (for a guide on fruit, please look up the Fructose Section in the "Diet" chapter).

Foods with a glycemic index above 55 are considered high glycemic index foods and include processed grains, sugar, starchy vegetables like potatoes, and sweet fruit like watermelon.

People with blood sugar issues are advised to limit foods with a glycemic index above 55, or combine the foods with a source of fat or protein, which slows down the ability of the food to increase blood sugar. Starchy carbohydrates that are converted quickly into glucose (such as pasta, bread, potato, white rice, banana) should be limited. Soda drinks should be completely avoided.

Fruits are a great source of vitamins and nutrients. However, in the initial phase of balancing blood sugar one should abstain from eating high glycemic index fruits, unless they are in combination with protein and/or fat. Low glycemic index fruit options should be eaten in preference.

Combining carbohydrates with protein can slow down the glycemic impact of the carbohydrates. A ratio of no larger than two servings of carbohydrate to one serving of protein should be consumed. For example, if you are having 4 grams of steak, you should have a maximum of 8 grams of potatoes.

Flaxseed and copper can help with balancing blood sugar.

Balancing Blood Sugar Rules

1) Include protein with every meal: eggs, nuts, seeds, fish, meat
2) Eat every two to three hours at first. Snacks are great!
3) No sweets before bed.
4) Avoid fruit juice.
5) Limit caffeine.
6) Avoid all grains and dairy, soy, corn, and yeast.
7) Eat breakfast within one hour of waking.
8) Include snacks rich in protein/fat every two to three hours.
9) No fasting.
10) Cut out foods with a glycemic index above 55.
11) Never skip breakfast.
12) Always combine carbohydrates with protein. Never exceed a 2:1 ratio of carb to protein.

Snacks

Some good snacks to consider may include: nuts, seeds, boiled eggs, homemade jerky, and protein shakes. Note: You may find that you are intolerant to some of these when you do the elimination diet, so do not invest in Costco-sized jugs just yet.

Rethink Your Breakfast

Typical SAD breakfast

Orange juice
Bagel with cream cheese
Coffee with sugar

Happy Breakfast

Eggs and Bacon
Herbal tea with Stevia
Grapefruit

Diabetes

Type II diabetes has been shown to result from lifestyle factors and has been previously described as progressive and chronic, however, recent advances have shown that it is reversible-by diet!

Type II diabetes used to predominately affect adults, but with our obesity epidemic, we are now seeing children as young as 8 developing this condition!. Our Western diet devoid of nutrients but full of junk is to blame. The usual treatment consists of a diabetic diet, oral medications, and insulin.

Diet effects on Type II diabetes have been well researched, but in recent years, alternative diets have been found to be much more effective than the Standard American "Diabetic Diet."

These diets can actually reverse diabetes, and not just prevent progression!

- Eight-week 600-calorie diet (semi-fasting)
- Low-carbohydrate diets
- Mediterranean
- Paleo Diet
- Vegetarian and vegan diets
- Native diets

All of these diets are low in refined grains and sugars (a.k.a. junk).

The 600-calorie diet can be dangerous, and is obviously not sustainable, most people will become diabetic once they go back to their old diets.

In contrast, low carbohydrate, Mediterranean, Paleo, vegetarian, vegan, and native diets can be quite tasty and are more akin to lifestyle change.

Dr. Mark Hyman has written "The Blood Sugar Solution," an excellent book on this topic.

Hashimoto's Carbohydrate Metabolism Abnormalities

Some people with Hashimoto's may not be able to tolerate any fruit or starchy vegetables, especially not at first. Up to 50% of people with Hashimoto's were found to have abnormalities in carbohydrate metabolism.

Following eating carbohydrates, blood sugar levels increase, which triggers insulin release to normalize blood sugar levels. Reactive hypoglycemia is an excessive release of insulin within four hours of eating carbohydrates that leads to low blood sugar levels.

Symptoms of low blood sugar may include: mental fog, blurry vision, sleeping difficulties, palpitations, fatigue, dizziness, sweating, headaches, depression, irritability, anxiety, sweet cravings, stuffy nose, panic attacks, numb/cold extremities, confusion, nausea, and hunger.

Low blood sugar levels are defined as <50 mg/dL, but some people may experience symptoms of low blood sugar at even higher levels. Normal fasting ranges of blood sugar vary between 70 and 100 mg/dL.

Adrenergic Postprandial Syndrome

When our blood sugar gets too low, we have a counter-regulatory response from our autonomic adrenergic system. Epinephrine and glucagon are released to counteract the low blood sugar when blood sugar reaches below 50 mg/dL. In people with adrenergic postprandial syndrome, epinephrine and glucagon may be released at higher blood sugar levels. People will experience the same unpleasant symptoms of hypoglycemia due to the epinephrine, but their actual blood sugar levels may come out normal.

Nighttime symptoms

A hypoglycemic state may also occur in the middle of the night. People may experience night sweats, nightmares and anxiety, or the person may not have any symptoms at all. This hypoglycemia will cause the adrenals to create more cortisol to raise the blood sugar back to normal, and cortisol will be depleted in the morning, leading to difficulty waking up. Drinking tea with coconut oil at bedtime may be helpful.

Treatment

The treatment for reactive hypoglycemia and postprandial syndrome consists of a low-carbohydrate diet with frequent smaller meals. Small meals should be added in the middle of the morning and the afternoon when blood sugar would start to decline.

A no-carbohydrate/low-carbohydrate diet was made popular by Dr. Robert Atkins, and in this type of diet, the body relies on fats instead of carbohydrates for energy. Breaking down fats keeps glucose levels much more stable compared with the breakdown of carbohydrates, and creates ketones.

Thus these diets are known as "Ketogenic diets." A ketogenic diet such as the Atkins diet may be helpful for reactive hypoglycemia, and has also been helpful in other conditions including mood disorders and epilepsy. Ketogenic diets generally limit carbohydrates from fruit, grains, and starches to fewer than 15 grams per day. Instead, they focus on meats, eggs, fats, and vegetables. Liberal amounts of coconut oil are also used with ketogenic diets. Coconut oil can be added to tea and sipped between meals. The classic ketogenic diet contains a 4:1 ratio by weight of fat to combined protein and carbohydrates.

As a caution, fasting diets and diets that are ultra-low carb may be helpful for healing in the short term, but may not be appropriate for everyone with thyroid issues, especially for a prolonged period.

Fasting and not enough carbohydrates can actually trigger the release of reverse T3, leading to those pesky hypothyroid symptoms in light of "normal" lab values.

Perhaps reverse T3 induces a "hibernation" state that helped us survive long winters as cavemen and women by preserving our metabolic function when we couldn't drive down to the market and only had limited amounts of food to eat.

Most people will report feeling energetic after starting a ketogenic diet, which may last from days to months, or even years for some. However, others, especially athletes and active individuals, may lose the energetic feeling and start to feel exhausted.

This is a sign that your body may need more carbohydrates. However, this does not mean that you should go back to eating pizza and soda three times a day! Keeping in mind blood sugar balancing rules, you can begin to add fruit, and if your gut healing is complete, incorporation of safe whole grains may be beneficial as well (quinoa, buckwheat, wild/brown rice), as you continue to nourish your body with organic meats, fats, and vegetables.

Caution for Vegans/Vegetarians

Recovering from adrenal fatigue and hypothyroidism when following a vegetarian diet is very challenging, as vegetarian diets are often carbohydrate heavy.

Vegetarian sources of protein such as legumes (beans), dairy, grains, soy and some seeds may be incompatible with trying to heal a leaky gut, which is almost always present with Hashimoto's. Pea protein is an alternative that may be easier to digest and is less likely to cause food sensitivities (I use NOW Foods brand).

Eggs, some seeds, and nuts would be the preferred sources of protein for vegetarians, however, some people with Hashimoto's may be intolerant to those as well, especially in the early stages of starting a healing diet.

Being a vegan is even more challenging, and nuts and seeds would be the go-to source of protein, which are usually too difficult to digest for many in the beginning of their thyroid healing journeys.

My Story

Before I was diagnosed with Hashimoto's, I was chronically stressed out. I would startle when someone walked into my office or almost jump out of my seat when my phone rang. I was an extremely light sleeper, every hum and squeak woke me up. I was full of nervous energy, my palms were sweaty, and my heart was always pounding. I felt cranky when I went without food for extended periods of time, and often lightheaded when I stood up. At first I thought that I must have suddenly developed a new onset anxiety disorder.

I also made a connection with my symptoms and the Sympathetic Nervous System (SNS). The SNS generated a fight-or-flight response in the presence of threatening situations. It was as though my fight-or-flight response was always turned on. I remember telling my mom; "My SNS is always on, it's overactive". Of course I now know that this activation becomes manifest when cortisol is depleted, as cortisol can no longer keep glucose levels up and the body starts experiencing hypoglycemic episodes (a.k.a. "Feed me or I will kill you!!").

Glycemic dysregulation was a big issue for me. I had a test that revealed that my insulin secretion was excessive in response to carbohydrates, and also had many symptoms of hypoglycemia, including palpitations, anxiety, fatigue, and night sweats after consuming sweets in the evening. Routine labs showed that my blood glucose levels were 53mg/dL (normal 70-110mg/dl) a few hours after eating a high-carb breakfast.

I now realize these fluctuations were leading to my anxiety. I felt so much better once I stabilized my blood sugar, and this has also resulted in a drop in antibodies. I limit my carbohydrate intake and stick to eating low-GI foods. Even too much fruit made me feel worse at first. I actually had to cut fruit out completely to start feeling better. I now incorporate plenty of coconut oil in my diet. I often put a tablespoon in herbal tea.

Stevia has been a wonderful replacement for the sugar I used to put in my tea.

Chapter Summary

✓ Adrenal dysfunction is closely related to thyroid dysfunction.
✓ Chronic stress leads to adrenal dysfunction, which results in hormone and nutrient depletion.
✓ DHEA is often low in autoimmune conditions.
✓ Addison's is full-blown adrenal failure and is often caused by an autoimmune condition.
✓ Inflammation and blood sugar imbalances contribute to adrenal dysfunction.
✓ Eating fat and protein with every meal and limiting carbohydrates helps to stabilize blood sugar and improve adrenal function.
✓ Vitamins (especially vitamin C), adaptogens, and PMG can be used to help recover adrenal function.
✓ Glandulars and hormones can be helpful but are associated with risks and should be used under the supervision of a knowledgeable health care professional.

"Healing is a matter of time, but it is sometimes also a matter of opportunity." ~Hippocrates

14: TRIGGERS

A variety of environmental triggers has been implicated in causing the development for Hashimoto's. We have already discussed how nutrient depletions, iodine excess, infections, adrenal dysfunction, and toxins can cause initial thyroid inflammation that sets off a vicious cycle when the immune system is imbalanced. The immune system becomes imbalanced in the presence of increased intestinal permeability, which seems to be the common thread between most autoimmune conditions.

Additional triggers that may contribute to Hashimoto's are hormonal imbalances, periodontitis, and viral triggers.

HORMONE IMBALANCES

Pregnancy

Pregnancy stimulates a shift from Th-1 to Th-2 dominance. This may explain why certain autoimmune conditions may go into remission during pregnancy, and why others are triggered by pregnancy.

As environmental/seasonal allergies are associated with Th-2 dominance, this explains why many women will report having increased allergies to pollens and other environmental allergies during pregnancy.

Tregs also increase during pregnancy to keep the immune system from attacking the developing fetus.

TPO and Tg antibodies decrease during pregnancy, reaching lowest levels during the third trimester, however, there is a rapid decrease in Tregs postpartum, resulting in a rebound of antibodies following delivery. Additionally TPOAb have been observed to increase six weeks postpartum, reaching previous levels at twelve weeks, and maximum levels twenty weeks post-delivery.

Pregnancy has also been identified as a trigger for autoimmune destruction of the thyroid. Some women have a transient postpartum autoimmune thyroid after giving birth, 80% of those women will spontaneously regain normal thyroid function, however, 20% will go on to develop Hashimoto's.

During pregnancy, fetal thyroid cells get into maternal thyroid cells. In some cases, these fetal cells can be found in the maternal thyroid for many years after the baby is born. There is a new theory that if the fetal cells persist after birth, this causes a host versus graft response, as the immune system is no longer suppressed by pregnancy Tregs and begins to recognize the fetal cells as foreign. However, this theory is still hypothetical, and has not been confirmed.

An alternate, more likely possibility is that nutrient depletion that occurs during pregnancy triggers thyroid inflammation. It is widely known that nutrient requirements increase during pregnancy, and pregnant women are advised to take prenatal vitamins. Women with TPO antibodies who supplemented selenium 200 mcg during pregnancy were found to have lower TPO antibodies during pregnancy and after giving birth compared with those who did not take selenium.

Additionally, only 28.6% of the selenium group developed postpartum thyroiditis compared with 48.6% of the group that did not take selenium.

Ultrasound monitoring showed that the thyroid appearance remained stable in the selenium group, while the group that did not take selenium showed thyroid tissue destruction.

Ideally, women should try to uncover their triggers before becoming pregnant, however this is not always realistic. Immune modulation is contraindicated during pregnancy, but adequate nutrition and perhaps selenium supplementation may improve outcomes. Thyroid hormone requirements also go up during pregnancy, thus close monitoring of thyroid function is recommend for those who are pregnant with Hashimoto's.

Oral Contraceptives

In addition to pregnancy, oral contraceptives (which produce a sort of "pseudo-pregnancy" due to the mix of hormones taken) stimulate a shift from Th-1 to Th-2. Similar changes in immune function may appear after stopping or starting oral contraceptives. As discussed in the "Depletions" chapter, oral contraceptives may cause depletions in our own endogenous hormones as well as in vitamins and minerals and beneficial bacteria.

But what are the alternatives for women who do not want to get pregnant? I had been using birth control pills for many years and knew I was not ready to get pregnant, but knew I had to kick the birth control habit. Condoms have a 14%-15% failure rate. That can be too big of a risk to take. I'm not too crazy about implants or any of the IUDs, either.

I then learned about the Fertility Awareness Method.

This method utilizes knowledge of the female reproductive cycle to predict days a woman will be fertile, and days that she isn't. There are only six days a woman can get pregnant within every cycle.

How birth control pills rob us of our health...(Blog Excerpt from www.thyroidrootcause.org) [1,2,3,4,5,6]

1. Birth control pills are described as "Drug Muggers" by Suzy Cohen, RPh, America's Pharmacist. Birth control pills deplete selenium, zinc and the amino acid tyrosine from our bodies. These are all nutrients that are necessary for proper thyroid function!

2. The hormones in birth control pills suppress our own body's production of estrogen and progesterone through a negative feedback loop mechanism. Birth control pills flood our bodies with high doses of artificial estrogen and progesterone leading our own production of natural hormones to turn off, preventing ovulation and thinning the uterine lining. This can lead to a hormonal imbalances such as estrogen dominance.

3. Birth control pills increase the risk of blood clots and strokes. The risk greatly increases after age 35 and for women who smoke.

4. Birth control pills can thin our bones leading to osteoporosis.

5. Oral contraceptives, which stimulate pseudopregnancy simulate a **shift from the Th1 to the Th2 Immune Branch.** This can produce an imbalance of the immune system perpetuating autoimmune conditions.

6. Birth control pills can change our normal flora, allowing yeast and other pathogenic organisms to thrive.

7. Women who take birth control pills have an altered preference to mates.

8. Birth control pills increase the risk of breast, ovarian and liver cancers.

9. Birth control pills impair our ability to build muscle despite exercise and can decrease sexual desire by suppressing testosterone (Yes, women produce small amounts of testosterone too).

11. High dose estrogen contained in birth control pills increases the activity of TBG (Thyroxine Binding Globulin). TGB binds thyroid hormone. More circulating TGB leads to lower levels of free thyroid hormone available for use by our body.

12. Many oral contraceptives contain lactose as an inactive filler. This may be an issue for many women with Hashimoto's who often present with

dairy and gluten intolerance issues.

13. Birth control pills lower our DHEA production. DHEA has been described as an anti-aging hormone. Many conditions, including autoimmune conditions have been associated with low DHEA.

14. Birth control pills deplete our bodies of folic acid, B_{12} and B_6 vitamins. A deficiency in any of these may result in anemia, birth defects, depression and other serious conditions....

With a typical menstrual cycle lasting twenty-eight days, (count day one as the first day of the menstrual period), on average, women ovulate somewhere in the middle. But not every woman has a twenty-eight-day cycle. Also, not every woman with a twenty-eight-day cycle ovulates right smack in the middle of the cycle. And many women may ovulate at different times each month depending on lifestyle factors.

Fertilization can occur five days before ovulation, or on the day of ovulation. Thus at the beginning and end of a menstrual cycle a woman will typically be infertile, and fertile for six days somewhere in the middle of the cycle.

A thermal shift in basal temperatures, cervical position, and cervical fluids help determine ovulation.

Our temperatures go up by 0.4-0.6 degrees Fahrenheit after ovulation, and this thermal shift can be measured by using a very sensitive basal thermometer right after waking up. The temperatures, along with the other fertility signs, are recorded daily in a fertility chart that will help the woman analyze where she is in the fertility cycle.

As a bonus, measuring basal temperatures can help with measuring progress in Hashimoto's treatment. Pre-ovulatory temperatures (usually the first ten to fifteen days of the cycle) indicate how well the thyroid and adrenals are performing.

A pre-ovulatory temperature is normally between 97.0 and 97.7 degrees Fahrenheit. Temps that are consistently lower than 97.3 degrees F may signal an underactive thyroid, while temps that are consistently above 97.7 degrees F may signal an overactive thyroid. Also, temperatures that are low but inconsistent, or all over the place, may signal adrenal insufficiency. You can document your interventions on the same fertility chart where you document the daily temperatures and fertility signs.

I highly recommend the book "Taking Charge of Your Fertility," which gives an amazingly descriptive and thorough overview of the Fertility Awareness Method for pregnancy prevention and achievement. After reading this book cover to cover, I have purchased a copy for all of my girlfriends!

While the Fertility Awareness Method can be very effective, I was still worried about doing it on my own. This method can fail in 25% of "typical" users, and I was afraid that I would fall into that category with my busy lifestyle.

That's when I found the Lady-Comp fertility monitor! This is a mini computer/alarm system that comes with an ultra-sensitive thermometer. This mini-computer learns your own body's normal temperatures and does the analysis for you, letting you know which days you are fertile with easy-to-read displays (red light=fertile, yellow light=learning, green light=infertile). If you are super-nerdy like me you can still make your own charts.

I have been using the Lady-Comp for over a year now, and it has been a really amazing tool that has taught me a great deal about my body. It has been an eye-opening experience watching my temperatures change, as well as noticing that all of a sudden my husband smelled really, really good after a jog around the time of my ovulation... (which is usually day seventeen or eighteen for me, not fourteen as some would lead you to believe).

According to the manufacturer "Lady-Comp is programmed with all natural family planning research data, it contains a database of more than 900,000 cycles and uses bio-mathematical forecasting calculations as well as the very latest computer techniques. It is a personal fertility monitor, which learns and adjusts to your individual cycle regardless of irregularities or cycle length. Several clinical studies confirm its 99.3% accuracy."

While this mini-computer is costly, fertility monitors are covered under Flex Spending and Health Spending accounts. Very good to know for those who "use it or lose it" at the end of the year, or want to plan for next year. It is also a onetime purchase. One month of brand-name birth control pills can cost upward of $100, thus the monitor pays for itself within a few months! (I included this last sentence for those of you who have husbands who work in finance, like mine does).

This monitor can also be used to plan a future pregnancy for when the time is right!

Of course, if the benefit of the oral contraceptives outweighs the risks, such as for certain serious medical conditions, a woman may need to continue taking the pill. In that case, supplementing with probiotics, magnesium, zinc, minerals, B vitamins, and vitamin C is strongly recommended.

FEMALE SEX HORMONES

Estrogen

Estrogen has been found to perpetuate inflammatory and autoimmune disease, while progesterone deficiency and estrogen fluctuations can worsen the autoimmune attack.

Estrogen appears to enhance Th-1 activity, whereas androgens (DHEA, testosterone) and progesterone suppress Th-1. A certain estrogen metabolite, known as 16α-hydroxyestrone (16α-OHE), has been implicated in proliferating autoimmune disease, and has been found in excess with those with autoimmunity.

Progesterone

Progesterone deficiency can surge into Th-1 dominance. This explains why the peak onset of Hashimoto's occurs during menopause, when the body's progesterone drops, or after pregnancy, when a rapid drop in progesterone occurs after the delivery.

Hormonal imbalances help to explain why women are affected by autoimmune conditions more often than men. Other substances, such as hormones in non-organic meats, endocrine-disrupting chemicals found in personal care products, and estrogenic activity of soy products can induce estrogen dominance and thus worsen or perpetuate autoimmunity.

Increasing fiber intake may also be helpful in eliminating excess circulating hormones.

Oftentimes, cutting out gluten, stabilizing blood sugar, proper nutrition, getting off birth control, and rebalancing the adrenals will rebalance estrogen and progesterone.

In other cases, however, more advanced strategies may need to be employed such as additional lifestyle interventions, additional supplements, or bio-identical hormones.

Many of the adrenal tests may be helpful in uncovering abnormalities in female hormones as well.

For a comprehensive book on lifestyle modifications, supplements and medications that can help rebalance female sex hormones, I highly recommend "The Hormone Cure" by Dr. Sara Gottfried.

PERIODONTITIS

Periodontitis is an inflammation of the gums that can lead to receding of the gums, loose teeth, and eventually tooth loss. Periodontitis is often found in Hashimoto's patients, and can be worsened by fluoride, the very substance added to our waters and toothpastes to prevent tooth decay.

The mechanism is as follows:
1) Buildup of plaque on the teeth from bacteria in the mouth.
2) Bacteria triggers an autoimmune response from the body, resulting in gum inflammation.

Symptoms
  ✓ Bleeding gums
  ✓ Puffy gums
  ✓ Receding gums
  ✓ Plaque buildup on teeth
  ✓ Loose teeth
  ✓ Bad breath

This bacterial imbalance in the mouth has been suggested to

contribute to Rheumatoid arthritis and Hashimoto's, and has been shown to increase IL-6, a Th-1 inflammatory marker in the body.

Changing our diet from a carbohydrate-based diet and starting fermented foods and probiotics will be helpful in rebalancing the bacteria, reducing the Gram-negative bacteria, and increasing the Gram-positive bacteria in both the mouth and the intestines.

Dr. Weston A. Price was a dentist who studied the effects of diet on dentition and found that those who ate traditional diets had far better teeth, and excellent health (no heart disease, autoimmune conditions, or obesity) compared with counterparts with similar genetic background who ate Western diets.

Gram-negative bacteria adhere to teeth and make it more difficult for saliva and brushing to get rid of them. Eating alkalizing foods, fermented foods, oil pulling and cranberry juice may be helpful for displacing the bacteria from teeth.

Oil pulling is an old Ayurvedic remedy of swishing around one tablespoon of sesame oil in the mouth, between the teeth, first thing in the morning for 5-20 minutes, until the oil turns white. In theory, this method helps to break down the "homes" of bacteria, which are usually made of microcapsules of oil. While water won't penetrate those microcapsules, sesame oil can, and mixes readily with the bacteria and becomes white in color. After 5-20 minutes the oil is spat out along with the toxins in it. Other oils have also been suggested to help, but sesame oil is the most commonly used.

Cranberry juice has been found to have anti-adhesion properties and is able to dissolve the protective coats that store the bacteria as well.

Doxycycline is an antibiotic that is used for periodontitis.

Interestingly, this same antibiotic has been reported to eliminate TPO antibodies for some, and may be an option to consider in someone with both Hashimoto's and periodontitis.

CHRONIC VIRAL INFECTIONS

Western lifestyle and autoimmune conditions

The "old friends hypothesis" proposed that Treg cells do not develop correctly because they are not exposed to parasites and other benign organisms that have co-existed with humans and co-evolved with us to "teach" our immune system how to evolve to threats.

In our modern-day world where we receive vaccines, use antibacterial soaps and take antibiotics, we are exposed far less to different bacteria, viruses, and parasites. This of course has many benefits, especially in the case of becoming affected with serious infections, however, it appears that we may also be missing out of some of these organisms that perhaps have had a beneficial effect on our immune system.

Autoimmune conditions and allergies are rare in Third-World countries that are plagued by parasites. This has led to another autoimmune theory, "The Hygiene Hypothesis." According to this theory, our immune system becomes "bored" as a result of not having enough parasites to get rid of, so instead it acts out against benign things like pollen and our own cells.

This theory is further supported by the suppression of certain autoimmune flares through the introduction of helminth (tapeworm) therapy. While I am not proposing that anyone give himself or herself a parasite in order to suppress their autoimmune condition, we need to consider the effects that certain substances can have in either promotion or suppression of autoimmunity.

Helminths have been found to be able to regulate various cytokines and downregulate inflammation, which is associated with the development of various autoimmune conditions.

The timing of infection may also matter as well, for example, children in developing countries usually contract the Epstein-Barr Virus when they are under the age of 10. This usually results in an asymptomatic infection—one that does not cause them symptoms. In contrast, in developed countries, where individuals are not usually exposed to the virus until they are in high school or college, the infection is symptomatic in 50% of the older kids affected. This is because by the time we reach college age, CD8+ T cells, the ones that fight EBV, have declined by threefold compared with the number of cells we had in childhood.

Overcoming Chronic viral infections

Some infections, like Yersinia, may be very easy to treat with antibiotics. Candida can be treated with an anti-candida diet and antifungal herbs and/or medications. Parasites can be treated with anti-parasitic medications and/or herbs.

However, Epstein-Barr, a virus, may be more challenging to treat with Western medicine. In its latent form, current anti-viral medications do not impact Epstein-Barr.

Viruses invade healthy host cells. As the viruses multiply inside of our cells, the cells burst, allowing the virus to infect additional cells. Thus, viruses are known as "intracellular" pathogens. A Th-1 response should be initiated in response to a virus, however, some viruses may trick our immune system.

Herpes viruses like EBV have been able to survive in our bodies by making proteins that suppress the Th-1 response. These proteins are similar to naturally occurring cytokines, and the body may not recognize that they are coming from the virus. The immune system does not make a strong enough Th-1 response, and the virus becomes concealed in our body, leading to a hidden chronic viral infection, and increasing the virus' chances of survival.

Many of us have been exposed to viral infections and thus have many dormant viruses that reside in our bodies. These viruses may live in harmony with the rest of the microbes, or they may be problematic.

Treating autoimmunity may be another approach to take when we are unable to go after individual infections.

A proposed approach would be to first normalize immune function through healing intestinal permeability, gut ecology, and supporting adrenal health, which will strengthen the immune system and help the body keep the opportunistic viruses, bacteria, fungi, and parasites under control instead of attacking them one at a time.

Additionally, animal fat and broths, soups and stews support the body's ability to suppress the viruses. Monolaurin/lauric acid, one of the components of coconut oil, has been found to be active against the Epstein-Barr virus. Replication of many viruses including Epstein-Barr is inhibited by glycyrrhizic acid, an active component of licorice root. Quercetin, Co-Enzyme Q10, N-Acetylcysteine, and glutathione were also reported to be helpful in chronic fatigue syndrome because of their anti-viral properties.

The amino acid Lysine at 4–6 grams per day can be helpful in supporting the immune system in controlling viral pathogens.

In contrast, Th-2 and potentially Treg stimulating substances may allow the virus to be more active. Eating citrus fruits, nuts, chocolate, coffee, and too many fresh fruits may allow the viruses to proliferate.

In many cases viral infections will learn to live in harmony with the rest of our bodies once the gut and adrenal function has been optimized. For EBV, optimizing Vitamin D levels and strengthening adrenals is very important.

Another hypothetical approach may be strengthening the Th-1 branch, as this would strengthen the virus killing immune response, however this can potentially worsen autoimmunity, and may be akin to cutting off your nose to spite your face!

Marshall Protocol

The Marshall Protocol, developed by Trevor Marshall Ph.D., is a multiyear treatment for autoimmune conditions of the Th-1 variety that includes pulsed doses of antibiotics, high doses of the blood pressure medication Benicar®, as well as the avoidance of vitamin D, sunlight, and soy for a period of one to five years.

Our immune system depends on vitamin D for proper immune system function. Dr. Marshall proposes that only endogenous vitamin D (1,25- dihydroxyvitamin-D), the kind produced by our bodies from cholesterol, is effective at modulating the immune system, and that vitamin D from the sun and supplements can be detrimental. According to Dr. Marshall's theory, supplemental vitamin D and its metabolites cause the immune system to function improperly. Additionally, pathogenic organisms can "hijack" the vitamin D receptor in our bodies, shutting down our vitamin D production.

The medication Benicar® is a vitamin D receptor agonist, and reactivates the vitamin D receptor to produce endogenous vitamin D that will correctly modulate the immune system. Measuring vitamin D levels before starting the protocol determines whether the person will benefit from the Marshall Protocol.

In 2008, it was reported that out of a cohort of twenty-four Hashimoto's patients who were undergoing the Marshall Protocol, seven of the nine patients improved in their first year of treatment, while two showed intermediate improvement. Three of five patients improved during the second year, and six out of the ten beyond their second year improved. Two patients did not improve in their second year of treatment, while a third did not improve beyond two years. The researchers were not certain whether these were treatment failures, or whether the patients needed longer treatment.

This approach may be useful for people whose autoimmune conditions were triggered by a viral infection.

However, I have many concerns regarding this treatment for Hashimoto's patients who often have adrenal fatigue and gut issues.

1) Adrenal fatigue results in low blood pressure, which can be worsened to dangerous levels with Benicar®, a medication used to reduce blood pressure.
2) More antibiotics can further cause gut dysbiosis.
3) People experience months to years of unpleasant die-off reactions
4) The protocol was originally designed for sarcoidosis, a different autoimmune condition with a unique profile.
5) The published results are questionable, citing "improvement" as an indicator instead of hard data like "TPO antibodies decreased," "TSH normalized," etc., that are usually measured in Hashimoto's.

I have not personally tried this protocol because of my conviction that an ancestral lifestyle that includes nutrient-dense foods and stress avoidance as well as plenty of sunlight is most complementary to our genes, and should be able to overcome most autoimmune conditions.

While the Marshall Protocol may seem like an interesting option for those with a viral Hashimoto's trigger, those who have not had an optimal response to the lifestyle modifications discussed in this book, or for those who may prefer to take medications and avoid sunlight instead of changing their diet, the results are not all that promising, and the protocol itself can be dangerous and must be done under the supervision of a trained clinician.

In addition to the triggers discussed in this book, there may be additional triggers that have not been identified yet. Perhaps you might discover that you have a unique trigger.

Chapter Summary

- ✓ Hormonal imbalances may trigger Hashimoto's.
- ✓ Selenium supplementation during pregnancy was helpful in preventing the occurrence of post-partum thyroiditis.
- ✓ Natural family planning methods can be helpful in kicking the birth control habit.
- ✓ Female sex hormones can contribute to immune imbalance but should normalize with proper care.
- ✓ Oil pulling, cranberry juice and doxycycline may be helpful for reducing detrimental bacteria in the mouth.
- ✓ Chronic viral infections hide out in our bodies in the dormant state.
- ✓ Strengthening the immune system may be helpful for overcoming Hashimoto's if triggered by chronic dormant infection.
- ✓ The Marshall Protocol is an alternative protocol for Th-1 dominant autoimmune conditions, but may be dangerous

"One man's food is another man's poison."

15: INTOLERANCES

A food intolerance is different from a food allergy. Although both types of reactions are mediated by the immune system, they are mediated by completely different mechanisms.

IgE Food Reaction

A food allergy is known as Type I Hypersensitivity, and is mediated by Immunoglobulin E (IgE), and manifests as hives, difficulty breathing, and is considered an immediate type of reaction. IgE allergies are also associated with allergies to medications like penicillin; bee stings, nut and shellfish allergies, as well as those pesky seasonal allergies we have to pollen and ragweed. The most accurate test for these types of allergies is a skin test, where an allergist will scratch the surface of the skin with the allergen, and observe for rashes, to see if the person is reactive to the substance. Blood tests are also available, but are less sensitive. This type of allergy is often called a "True Allergy" by medical professionals.

However, this terminology is a misnomer, and suggests that only IgE allergies exist, and that reactions mediated by different parts of the immune system are nonexistent. Challenge any of your medical professionals to look back into their Immunology notes and they will find that there are additional types of hypersensitivities that are just as "true" and "real" as IgE anaphylactic reactions. The two relevant hypersensitivities are mediated by immunoglobulins A and G, IgA and IgG, respectively.

For lack of better terminology, IgA and IgG hypersensitivities have both been labeled as "food intolerance" or "food sensitivity," however, they are much different in their mechanism and propensity to cause harm in the body.

IgA Food Reactions (Celiac-like)

IgA food intolerance is the more severe reaction and works primarily in the intestines. It is an abnormal response of the intestines to certain foods in genetically predisposed individuals. The intolerances may manifest themselves early in childhood, or later in life.

IgA food intolerance results in irritation and inflammation of the intestinal tract every time that particular food is consumed. This results in damage to the intestines, with an eventual inability to absorb nutrients, and can increase the risk of autoimmune diseases, cancer, and accelerate aging through increased intestinal permeability.

IgA food intolerances may be asymptomatic, or they may present with the following symptoms: diarrhea, loose stools, constipation, acid reflux, malabsorption of nutrients from foods, and increased intestinal permeability.

They may cause IBS, gas, nausea, skin rashes (including eczema), acne, respiratory conditions such as asthma, nasal congestion, headache, irritability, and vitamin/mineral deficiencies.

The most well-known IgA food reaction has been called "celiac" disease, and it is an intolerance to gluten, the protein found in wheat. However, dairy protein, egg, and soy protein IgA intolerances are also extremely common in those with Hashimoto's. These IgA food intolerances do not have a specific name, and are often confused with other, less severe food absorption syndromes.

For example, when I told my well-educated pharmacist friend that I had a dairy intolerance, she said "Oh, I'm lactose intolerant too. Can't you just take Lactaid®?"

Of course, lactose intolerance and dairy protein intolerance are two completely different things. Lactose is a milk sugar, and the ability to digest lactose depends on having an enzyme named "lactase," or intestinal bacteria that digest the milk sugar. Lactose intolerance can cause bloating, diarrhea, etc., but does not cause intestinal tissue inflammation or damage.

A more accurate description of an IgA food reaction may be Protein-Mediated Autoimmune Intestinal Inflammatory Reaction (PAIR).

Table 11: Protein-Mediated Autoimmune Intestinal Inflammatory Reactions

Food	Reactive Proteins
Wheat, rye, barley	Gluten
Dairy	Casein, whey (alpha and beta lactoalbumins)
Eggs	Ovo-albumin
Soy	

People with Hashimoto's may have one or multiple PAIR intolerances, but be clueless of the effect of these substances on their well-being. This is because the reactions may not always be immediate, and over time, as we continue eating these foods, the body will have a dull response to them. Eliminating the foods for a period of time, following by a re-challenge will unmask the response. Lifelong avoidance of PAIRs may be necessary for most people, however, some people have been able to reintroduce these foods after following programs like the GAPS diet/SCD Diet for one to two years.

Lab testing for PAIR intolerances is done through an IgA test. IgA is a type of antibody that is secreted in the intestines. This can be done as a blood test or saliva test. The four most common PAIRs are to gluten, dairy, eggs, or soy. Many physicians are not aware of these types of tests, and will instead order IgE tests, which will obviously not show an intestinal reaction.

Some professionals believe that removing food intolerances, especially eggs, dairy, soy, and gluten, will lead to the reversal of the autoimmune condition, by helping heal intestinal permeability.

In many cases eliminating these foods will work. There have been many reported cases of the disappearance of TPO antibodies after three to six months on a gluten-free diet. Other individuals have reported the reversal of autoimmune thyroiditis by removing dairy from the diet. Others removed eggs, soy, or all four PAIRs in order to reverse their autoimmune condition.

IgG Food Reactions

In the presence of increased intestinal permeability, food particles enter the blood through the "loosened" tight junctions, and the body will develop IgG antibodies to these foods. These are the same kind of antibodies formed to thyroid tissues. As intestinal permeability is always present in autoimmune conditions, most people with Hashimoto's will have multiple IgG food reactions, often to the foods they eat most frequently.

Reactive foods seem to perpetuate the autoimmune thyroid reaction. The presence of IgG4 subtype antibodies (type that occur to foods) seem to correlate with the amount of thyroid damage.

Leaky gut was observed in 50% of patients with food intolerance.

Furthermore, food intolerances increase intestinal permeability, thus creating a vicious self-perpetuating cycle. Studies showed that withdrawal of the foods that caused intolerance for six months did not reverse the leaky gut, so while removing triggering foods is an important first step, it won't completely solve the problem as food intolerances seem to develop as a result of leaky gut and perpetuate it, but do not cause it.

IgG intolerances are also known as delayed type intolerances that may take up to a few days to manifest. These intolerances may cause systemic inflammation and perpetuate intestinal permeability. Although IgG food intolerances haven't been studied as well as the other types of food reactions, research suggests that they may be associated with a multitude of symptoms such as gastrointestinal disturbances, migraine headaches, drowsiness, and discomfort.

Some professionals believe that these intolerances are specifically associated with intestinal permeability, and that any food eaten excessively will result in an IgG reaction, in the presence of intestinal permeability. Instead of removing these foods completely, they recommend removing them for a short period (three to six months) and then rotating them every four to seven days while working on healing intestinal permeability. Once the intestinal permeability resolves, so should the IgG reactions.

In my experience, IgG tests may be helpful to pinpoint the foods that may be causing additional reactions, which may need to be removed or rotated short-term.

Unfortunately for most, removing IgG food intolerances may only be a temporary fix, if intestinal permeability is not addressed. You may remove the foods that were positive on IgG antibody tests, only to find that a month later you have become sensitive to more foods.

Dr. Natasha Campbell-McBride, creator of the GAPS diet, cautions that the intestines of those with Hashimoto's are like sieves, and that patients with Hashimoto's may often present with multiple IgG reactions. She explains that intestinal permeability causes the food intolerances and that eliminating the offending foods will only help temporarily if leaky gut is not addressed, as the person will develop new intolerances, usually to the foods eaten most commonly.

Thus, the leaky gut is the root cause of the problem, not the food intolerance. Dr. Campbell-McBride advises focusing on healing intestinal permeability to resolve IgG type intolerances.

In most cases of intestinal permeability, a rotation diet may need to be started for remaining foods to prevent from getting new reactions to the foods. Foods are rotated in every 4-7 days and never eaten two days in a row.

IgG tests are available as panels of 100–200 foods and may be helpful in identifying additional intolerances that can cause an immune system response. However, these tests are somewhat controversial, and may have false negatives to the foods that people eat most often.

Other Foods Associated with Autoimmunity

The most common food antigens that account for 90% of food reactions are milk, eggs, peanuts, tree nuts (such as almonds, cashews, walnuts), fish, shellfish, soy, and wheat.

Nightshades (found in tomatoes, potatoes, peppers, and eggplant), as well as beef, citrus, corn and pork may also be problematic.

As we have already discussed, PAIRs are a factor present in most cases of autoimmunity, especially in Hashimoto's.

Gluten has been the most well-researched PAIR, and it seems to cause an increase in intestinal permeability in everyone, not just those who have a genetic susceptibility to gluten sensitivity. In some, removal of gluten will lead to intestinal healing within three months, in others, it may take up to two years. Other foods may cross-react with gluten and cause a similar immune response as well as intestinal permeability, and include: dairy products, chocolate, yeast, oats, and coffee.

When people cut gluten out of their diet, they may begin to rely more heavily on gluten-free grains like quinoa, rice, amaranth, etc., which can be problematic if they continue to have intestinal permeability, as they may be more difficult to digest. Grains require brush border enzymes for digestion, and in advanced cases of PAIRs, the brush borders may be severely impaired. Grains and other starchy foods may need to be removed until the gut has healed include: sesame, buckwheat, sorghum, millet, hemp, amaranth, quinoa, tapioca, teff, corn, rice, and potato.

IgA and IgG tests can be helpful and a good guide for where to start. I never would have guessed I had a reaction to dairy (IgA) pineapple (IgG), peach (IgG), or watermelon (IgG). But they are not affordable for everyone. Additionally, while labs are available to test for the four most common PAIRs, they may show false negatives and people may have a PAIRs reaction to foods that are not available as IgA tests. Thus, some professionals still recommend following an elimination diet, even if the test results for PAIRs and IgG intolerances were negative. I have also had success with ALCAT testing.

Other professionals do not use lab tests at all, and simply have their patients follow an elimination diet, which is considered the gold standard for identifying food intolerances.

ELIMINATION DIETS

In contrast to other diets that simply exclude common problematic foods, an elimination diet is done to determine which particular food intolerances the individual may have.

When we eat the foods that our body is sensitive to on a daily basis, it is very difficult to connect the foods with the symptoms we are having. For example, people who have a dairy sensitivity but continue to eat dairy multiple times a day might be tired, have joint pain, congestion, bloating, and acid reflux on daily basis, but won't be able to pinpoint the symptom to the foods.

This is because every time we eat this food, the body becomes depleted in its ability to protect itself from the antigenic food, and the reactions become less specific and more chronic. If the food continues to be given, the body will become sensitive to more and more things.

Once the sensitizing food is eliminated for a few days to a few weeks, the person should generally feel better and experience less bloating, less reflux, normal bowel movements, more energy, etc.

When the person is exposed to the food again, the body will actually produce a stronger, more specific reaction, allowing the person to recognize which particular food is problematic to him/her.

Some symptoms that may occur when one is exposed to a sensitizing food include gastrointestinal symptoms such as diarrhea, bloating, acid reflux, burning, gas, or cramping. Respiratory, muscular, and skin symptoms may be seen as well. Please consult Table 12 on the next page for some of the symptoms experienced.

TABLE 12: COMMON FOOD SENSITIVITY SYMPTOMS

System	Symptoms
Respiratory	Postnasal drip, congestion, cough, asthma symptoms
Gastrointestinal	Constipation, diarrhea, cramping, bloating, nausea, gas, acid reflux, burning, burping
Cardiovascular	Increased pulse, palpitations
Skin	Acne, eczema, itchiness
Muscular	Join aches, pain, swelling, tingling, numbness
Mental	Headache, dizziness, brain fog, anxiety, depression, fatigue, insomnia

There are a few different ways that elimination diets can be done. We will discuss a basic elimination diet and an advanced elimination diet.

Basic Elimination Diet

A basic elimination diet takes out the most antigenic foods for three weeks and allows most gluten-free grains (except corn).

A diet clean of reactive foods should be followed for three weeks, and should at least remove the top eight antigenic foods: gluten, dairy, soy, eggs, corn, nuts, shellfish, preservatives, and possibly Nightshades, caffeine, alcohol, legumes, citrus fruits, fructose, grains, and tubers such as potatoes.

After three weeks, foods will be introduced one by one, every three days, to help unmask hidden food reactions.

Figure 14: Basic Elimination Diet

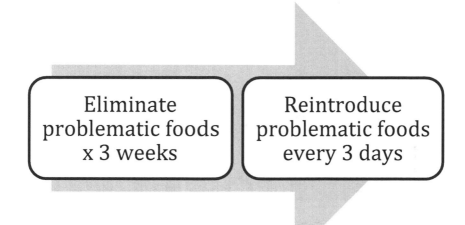

Eliminate problematic foods x 3 weeks

Reintroduce problematic foods every 3 days

Most Problematic Foods, for Elimination
1. Gluten
2. Dairy
3. Soy
4. Eggs
5. Corn
6. Nuts
7. Shellfish
8. Preservatives

Table 13: Basic Elimination Diet Sample Meal Plan

Breakfast	buckwheat and banana
Lunch	quinoa, chicken breast, and avocado salad
Dinner	salmon, rice and beans, steamed carrots, zucchini, broccoli
Snack	pumpkin seeds and apple

Reintroduction Schedule
1) Nuts
2) Corn
3) Eggs
4) Soy
5) Dairy
6) Gluten

SAMPLE FOOD INTRODUCTION JOURNAL

Date	Food Introduced	My Symptoms
3/1/12	Dairy	Joint pain, tingling, stomach pain
3/4/12	Eggs	Gas, bloating

Advanced Elimination Diet

An advanced elimination diet that combines food elimination with healing may be more appropriate for Hashimoto's patients with multiple food intolerances and more gastrointestinal symptoms, or ones who continue to have symptoms after following a basic elimination diet.

I developed this diet after cutting out all tested food intolerances, (including gluten, dairy, and soy) for one year only to start having bloating and new food intolerances (almonds, eggs, bananas).

It may be best to do the more extreme version of the elimination diet rather than leaving things in and being sorry later.

The three-week elimination diet can be done by combining the elemental diet with a healing phase, similar to the one recommended by the GAPS diet.

New foods should be introduced every three days, starting with the ones that are well-cooked and easiest to digest.

We start with bone and meat broths with well-cooked meats and vegetables that are pureed, and gradually introduce more solid foods while we continue the healing broths.

The diet can be jump-started with an elemental diet for one to seven days that will allow the digestive system and intestines to rest and regenerate.

This diet is akin to a "baby food diet," or a diet that one would use to introduce new foods to a baby. This is because like babies' intestines, the intestines of many Hashimoto's patients are permeable.

Figure 15: Advanced Healing/Elimination Diet

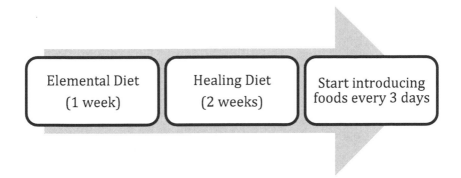

In addition to excluding foods that are detrimental, we include healing foods to help the body regenerate.

Foods Recommended for Autoimmune Thyroid Healing
1) Bone and meat broths
2) Gelatin
3) Protein
4) Liver
5) Meat
6) Saturated fat
7) Fermented foods
8) Probiotics
9) Vegetable juices (fiber removed)
10) Well cooked vegetables, pureed vegetables

Sample Introduction Diet (Days One to Three)

Breakfast	Chicken stock, chicken meat, pureed zucchini
Lunch	Chicken stock, chicken meat, pureed carrots
Dinner	Chicken stock, chicken meat, pureed zucchini
Snack	Chicken stock, chicken meat, pureed carrots

Introduction Schedule

Fiber is limited in the first two to four weeks, allowing for the intestinal lining to heal. Potentially reactive foods are introduced every three days, starting with eggs, which are introduced after three weeks and continued if there is no reaction.

Grains, dairy, beans, and legumes are excluded for the first ninety days. The goal of this diet is to heal the intestinal lining, allowing the body to have fewer food reactions, so if a particular food is not tolerated at first, the healing diet is continued and the food is reattempted in one month.

For more guidance and proposed meal plans, recipes, and food journals for the Advanced Healing/Elimination diet, go to www.thyroidrootcause.org/guide

Supplements

Protein molecules are the most difficult to digest of all foods. Their digestion is a multi-step process, starting with the stomach and the gastric enzyme pepsin (discussed in the Digestion & Depletions chapter).

Additionally, proteins are further broken down by proteolytic enzymes secreted by the pancreas. The pancreas releases enzyme precursors that need to become activated by enterokinase, an enzyme secreted by the small intestine to finish the final step of protein digestion- conversion of proteins into free amino acids. Due to SIBO and other issues affecting the small intestine, these enzymes do not become activated in many individuals with Hashimoto's.

Proteolytic enzyme supplements (sometimes called "systemic

enzymes" provide the activated enzymes (protease blends, trypsin, chymotrypsin, elastase, carboxypeptidase) and should be taken between meals and help to break down circulating immune complexes formed by poorly digested proteins, and may be helpful in reducing TPO Antibodies.

Chapter Summary

✓ Food intolerances are distinct from food allergies and are mediated by different parts of the immune system (IgG, IgA).
✓ Due to increased intestinal permeability, people with Hashimoto's also have food intolerances.
✓ Food intolerances exacerbate autoimmunity by perpetuating intestinal permeability and possibly cross-react with thyroid antibodies.
✓ The most common antigenic substances are dairy, eggs, gluten and soy.
✓ Testing for food intolerances is available.
✓ Elimination diets are the most helpful in finding foods that are problematic for each individual.
✓ Consider proteolytic enzymes to help reduce circulating immune complexes.

My Story

I was personally shocked to find out that I had an IgA milk protein (casein) intolerance. I consumed dairy products two or three times a day for many years. I also had severe bloating and acid reflux, but never connected the two. I was amazed at how flat my stomach felt and how my symptoms disappeared after three days of going dairy free. If I accidentally have a casein product now, I feel a burning sensation in my intestines, which is followed by tingling in my extremities and painful diarrhea.

"The best way to detoxify is to stop putting toxic things into the body and depend upon it's own mechanisms". ~Andrew Weil, MD

16: TOXINS

We are bombarded by toxins in our environment every day, from the air we breathe, the water we drink, the food we consume and the products we use. Some of us may not be able to detoxify our bodies leading to a perpetuation of autoimmunity.

In 2006, the Centers for Disease Control reported that the average American has 116 out of 148 synthetic compounds in his or her body, including dioxins, polycyclic hydrocarbons, and organochloride pesticides. This is especially significant for those who want to get pregnant. The average umbilical cord contains 217 neurotoxins, 208 of which are known to cause birth defects.

We now have more than 80,000 different chemicals, and many of them have not been evaluated for human safety, yet we encounter them daily. There are too many to discuss in this book, but more information can be found on www.ewg.org, the consumer website of the Environmental Working Group, a U.S. environmental health research and advocacy organization. We will discuss a few well-known chemicals that are prevalent in everyday life and may be detrimental to people with Hashimoto's.

ENDOCRINE DISRUPTORS IN YOUR HOME

Endocrine disruptors are chemicals that interfere with our hormones. Some of these chemicals may affect thyroid activity, some mimic estrogen, while others may cause cancerous tumors, birth defects, and developmental disabilities.

HALOGENS

The halogens bromide, chloride, and fluoride compete with iodine for the receptor binding sites in the thyroid, but instead of activating the receptors they build up in thyroid tissue and cause thyroid cell death and inflammation. Studies have shown that individuals exposed to a variety of halogen-containing substances had a high incidence of TPO antibodies.

These substances were studied in the industrial world, where exposed workers showed a trend in increased incidence of Hashimoto's. Unfortunately, they are commonly found in consumer products as well.

Fluoride

Most U.S. communities began to add fluoride to the drinking water in an effort to prevent tooth decay, starting in 1945. While various studies have shown that fluoride reduces the incidence of dental cavities and tooth decay, fluoride is an endocrine disruptor and studies confirm that fluoride is directly toxic to thyroid cells and causes thyroid cell death, suppressing thyroid activity.

In fact, fluoride was used to treat hyperthyroidism up until the 1950s, prior to the development of other thyroid-suppressing medications. Fluoride is effective as a thyroid suppressor at doses of 0.9-4.2 mg per day for hyperthyroidism. Most adults in fluoridated communities are ingesting between 1.6 and 6.6 mg of fluoride per day from water inadvertently suppressing their thyroid function.

Studies from China, India, and Russia have shown a reduction in T3 and an increase in TSH in those exposed to fluoride in the workplace or through drinking water. We know that whenever TSH increases, more TPO is released leading to the release of hydrogen peroxide (H_2O_2). Hydrogen peroxide damages the thyroid cells in the absence of enough selenium and glutathione. This triggers a stress response from the cells, leading to accumulation of white blood cells and resultant inflammation. In those with increased intestinal permeability, this inflammation becomes permanent and thyroid antibodies develop.

Another Government-Induced Disease?

Dr. Weston A. Price, a dentist, traveled around the world photographing the teeth of various cultures. He found that those who ate a traditional diet had perfect arches and no cavities. In contrast, those who adopted a "modern" diet containing flour, sugar, and processed vegetable fats began to have improper jaw development, resulting in crowding of teeth, as well as tooth decay.

Fluoridation partially began as a collaborative effort between dental associations, the U.S. government and sugar lobbyists who wanted to find a solution that would allow people to have fewer cavities while continuing to consume just as much sugar. Proper nutrition should be emphasized and should eliminate the need for fluoride.

Just like other halogens, fluoride may act as a trigger in inducing thyroid cell death and inflammation and leading to the development of thyroiditis/autoimmune thyroiditis.

The United States is one of the only countries that adds fluoride to the water system. In fact, 97% of European countries have rejected water fluoridation due to the toxicity associated with it. However, Austria, France, Germany, Spain, and Switzerland allow the addition of fluoride to salt.

Some people have reported improvement in thyroid symptoms and thyroid function tests following removing fluoride from their lifestyle.

Common sources of fluoride

- Supplements (check the labels)
- Bottled beverages
- Toothpaste
- Black tea
- Red tea
- Canned food items
- Black/red rock salt
- Chewing tobacco
- Medications

Doggie Hashimoto's

Dogs, our sweet companions, have been found to have a high incidence of autoimmune thyroiditis, similar to Hashimoto's.

The Environmental Working Group has found that commercial dog food has a very high level of fluoride.

Additionally, while wolves in the wild don't typically eat grain products, dog foods contain a high amount of wheat and gluten.

Perhaps the combination of fluoride and gluten in dog food (as well as fluoride in Fido's water) deserves further attention.

Tea

Boiling water concentrates the fluoride instead of getting rid of it, while freezing the water does not affect the concentration of fluoride.

Fluoride is also found in tea, especially red and black tea. Tea leaves accumulate fluoride from the soil and pollution. The longer they stay on the tea tree, the heavier the fluoride content. An article published in the journal Food and Chemical Toxicology said there is up to 4.5, 1.8 and 0.5 mg/L of fluoride in black, green and white teas, respectively, when brewed for five minutes. Chamomile and herbal tea contained 0.13 mg/L.

Fluoride-Containing Medications

Fluoride-containing medications include anesthetics, antacids, anti-anxiety medications, antibiotics, antidepressants, anti-fungals, anti-histamines, cholesterol-lowering medications, anti-malarial medications, chemotherapy, appetite suppressants, arthritis medications, psychotropics, and steroids.

Some of the most commonly used medications that contain fluoride include:

- Prozac®, Lexapro®, Celexa®, Paxil®: used for depression, anxiety, or obsessive-compulsive disorder
- Prevacid®: used for acid reflux
- Diflucan®: an antifungal used for yeast infections.
- Fluoroquinolone antibiotics (Cipro®, Levaquin®, Avelox®): used for UTIs and other infections
- Celebrex®: used for pain
- Lipitor®, Zetia®: used to lower cholesterol

Full list at http://www.slweb.org/ftrcfluorinatedpharm.html

Filters

Fluoride can be taken out by distilling the water, reverse osmosis filtration systems, and activated alumina defluoridation filters. Most other filters do not remove fluoride. Exchanging black and red tea for white tea or herbal tea may be helpful as well.

Substances containing two other halogens—chlorine and bromine—have also been found to induce autoimmune thyroiditis.

Bromide

Studies have shown that bromide-containing substances, polybrominated diphenylethers (PBDEs) are connected to an increased incidence of Hashimoto's. Bromide is found in baked goods, plastics, soft drinks, and tea, as well as in our mattresses, which now contain brominated flame retardants. This is a "safety feature" instituted by the U.S. government to prevent mattresses from rapidly bursting into flames from cigarettes as someone falls asleep while smoking in bed. Great help for the minority who like to smoke in bed, but not so much for health-conscious people who do not smoke.

PBDEs are also frequently found in furniture foam and plastics used in computers, appliances, and electronic products. Over time, PBDEs can leach from these products and get into the environment.

Chlorine

Chlorine containing polychlorinated biphenyls (PCBs) have been shown to be toxic to thyroid cells and promote the onset of Hashimoto's Thyroiditis. Studies have shown that PCBs increase

TSH, thyroid autoantibodies, and thyroid size. In addition to industrial products, chlorine is found in water systems, pools, cleaning products, and plastics. Additionally, it is found in the crop pesticide organochlorine, which accelerates thyroid hormone elimination and can play a role in autoimmunity.

XENOESTROGENS

Xenoestrogens are endocrine-disrupting chemicals that mimic the effects of estrogen and include soy, BPA, phthalates, and parabens. The continued use and accumulation of these substances may lead to estrogen dominance and can have a profound impact on the immune system, adrenal, and thyroid function, as well as cause birth defects, infertility, and cancers.

Soy isoflavones are found in many processed foods as well as some supplements. Always be sure to read your food and vitamin packaging. Better yet, avoid all processed food like the plague!

BPA (bisphenol-A) is found in plastics such as containers, baby formula cans, as well as store register receipts, which are coated in BPA. BPA has been linked to cancers, reproductive disorders, as well as developmental disorders. BPA also antagonizes T3 receptors, essentially shutting them down. You should look for "BPA-free" plastic products, or better yet, avoid cooking or storing your food in plastics.

Phthalates are found in many detergents, laundry products, and washable items. In addition, they are found in cosmetics, plastics, moisturizers, soaps, house paint, and perfumes. Phthalates have been implicated in cancers, endocrine disruption, diabetes and obesity. They may be listed on the packaging of products (such as diethyl phthalate), or they may be disguised under the word "fragrance".

Check the ingredient list of your beauty products and only use those that do not contain dibutyl phthalate (DBP). Avoid using personal care products, detergents, and cleansers that contain "fragrance" in the ingredient list—"fragrance" commonly includes diethyl phthalate (DEP).

Triclosan is found in antibacterial soaps, deodorants, hairsprays, and toothpastes. The structure of triclosan resembles the structure of thyroid hormones, and it has been associated with altered levels of thyroid hormone in animals. Avoid the use of "antibacterial" products. They are not necessary in the home. If you need to use an antimicrobial product for work or disinfecting purposes, use an alcohol hand rub or rinse product that does not list triclosan or "fragrance" in the ingredients.

Parabens are found in body washes, shampoos, and lotions and are used as microbial agents. They have been implicated in breast cancers and with causing skin reactions. Look for the ending "paraben" as in methylparaben in your personal care products. Choose products that do not list parabens in the ingredients.

Better Living Through Chemistry?

Much controversy has come from the advertisements we watch on television and see in magazines that make us think we are inadequate, unattractive, dirty, and flawed. Teenage girls are especially susceptible, and glossy magazines with pictures of airbrushed models have been blamed for eating disorders and self-esteem issues in young women.

Looking into an average American woman's bathroom, you will likely find close to 100 personal care products: Nail polish, lotion, shampoo, make-up remover, eyeliner, face masks, hair spray,

Table 14: Partial List of Environmental Agents That Interfere with Thyroid Function

Agent	Example of Sources	Mode of Action	Human Studies
PCBs*	Found in coolants and lubricants	Thyroid receptor agonist/antagonist, can alter levels of T4 and TSH	Increase in TSH, thyroid volume, thyroid antibodies
Organochlorine pesticides	Used as pesticide on crops	Accelerates metabolism of T4	No human studies
PBDEs*	Found in flame retardants	Bind to thyroid receptors, displaces T4 from binding proteins	Increase in Hashimoto's.
BPA	Used in plastic bottles	Antagonizes thyroid receptors	No human studies
Perchlorate, thiocyanate	Rocket fuel, fertilizer, smoking	Inhibits iodine uptake	No human studies
Triclosan	Antibacterial in soaps	Reduce serum T4	No human studies
Isoflavones*	Soy products	Inhibits TPO activity	Potential increase in Hashimoto's

Adapted from Eschler DC, Hasham A, Tomer Y. Cutting edge: The etiology of autoimmune thyroid diseases. Clin Rev Allergy Immunol.2011 October; 41(2): 190-197

*Human studies have associated as a trigger or accelerator in development of Hashimoto's.

perfume, the list goes on and on. These products are full of chemicals that have not had safety studies done to verify that they are non-toxic to humans. Most cosmetic chemists only test the chemicals on themselves to see if the products make them more aesthetically appealing for one reason or another. Laboratory tests to access blood levels, changes in organ or immune system function; or any other available medical tests are not a practice followed by the cosmetic industry.

You may think that only the things you eat matter, but in fact, the skin is an excellent delivery system for chemicals. Many topical patches and creams are used to deliver pharmaceuticals and hormones directly into the blood stream (think Ortho Evra® birth control patch).

Products that are swallowed are usually worked on by the liver to make them less toxic before they go into circulation. This is known as first pass-effect, and only a small percentage of the original product may get into the circulation. In contrast, products applied to the skin actually bypass the liver and go directly into the circulation, and can produce systemic effects until they get to the liver to be eliminated. Dr. Nicholas Perricone, the well-known anti-aging dermatologist, reports that many facial creams, lotions, and serums marketed to women actually contain estrogens.

In contrast, men generally use much fewer personal care products, so perhaps women's routine use of endocrine-disrupting products leads to the disproportionate female predominance of thyroid and autoimmune conditions. The use of lipstick, in particular, has been connected to the development of lupus, an autoimmune condition.

What To Do?

Go on a make-up, perfume, and body wash holiday! You can also choose products that are more natural in their origins. One rule to follow: if you wouldn't eat it, don't put it on your body. The EWG website hosts a database of thousands of personal care products, each with its own safety rating based on dozens of toxicity and regulatory databases, Skin Deep.

Once you realize that the TV commercials, magazines, and Internet ads are programming you to consume more and more without taking your health, happiness, or well-being into account, you will think twice about what you put in your home, in your body, or on your skin.

What's Hiding In Your Bathroom?

Avoid the following ingredients in your personal care products/cosmetics.

Type of Product	Ingredients to Avoid
Bar soap	Triclocarban
Liquid soap	Triclosan
Moisturizers, lotions	Retinyl palmitate, retinol
Toothpaste	Triclosan
Lip glosses and lipsticks	Retinyl palmitate, retinol
Shampoo and conditioner	Fragrance, PEG, ceteareth, polyethylene, parabens: (such as propyl paraben), DMDM hydantoin
Nails	Formaldehyde, formalin, toluene, dibutyl phthalate
Sunscreen	Retinyl palmitate, oxybenzenone

Other Toxic Chemicals

Other toxins that may not have specific effect on thyroid function, but can burden the body's ability to detoxify and heal itself, include dioxins, which are found in bleached paper products. Tampons are especially problematic as they can be absorbed through the vaginal membranes into circulation. Chemicals used in dry cleaning are extremely toxic and have been associated with an increased risk of cancer. Also, conventional cleaning supplies used to clean our bathrooms, kitchens, and floors are full of toxic chemicals. You can make your own cleaning supplies or purchase ones that are made from natural ingredients. The EWG has a database of safer, cleaner alternatives: http://www.ewg.org/guides/cleaners

Non-toxic alternatives for cleaning

1) Baking soda: makes water soft, increases cleaning capacity of soap, good for scrubbing
2) Borax: cleans and removes odors, excellent disinfectant
3) Soap from plants: nontoxic and biodegradable. Available as liquid, flakes, and bars, the best are without synthetic additives, flavors, and colors.
4) Vinegar: cleans grease and limestone residue
5) Citric acid and lemon: removes grease, limestone residue, and refreshes
6) Natural essential oils: natural extracts and essential oils enhance antibacterial and antiviral properties of cleaning products. Antibacterial: camphor, cardamom, citronella, cypress, eucalyptus, ginger, juniper, lavender, lime, lemongrass, orange, lemon, pine, rosemary, sage, sandalwood, tea tree, thyme. Antiviral: cinnamon, eucalyptus, lavender, lemon, oregano, sandalwood, tea tree.

Mom's Cleaning Recipes

Dishwashing Liquid	Glass Cleaner
Juice from 3 lemons 1 ½ cup of water 1 cup of salt 1 cup vinegar Mix and boil for 10 min. while stirring, until liquid thickens. Pour into glass container while still warm	1/4 cup white vinegar 1 tablespoon cornstarch 1 quart warm water Add to spray bottle, wipe with crumpled newspaper
Sink Cleaner	**Garbage Disposal**
1/3 cup baking soda warm water to make into paste Use on a sponge to scrub	Grind half of a lemon to clean and freshen
Toilet Cleaner	**Ceramic Floor Tiles**
¼ cup of baking soda 1 teaspoon vinegar Pour into toilet bowl, leave for ½ hour, wipe and flush	¼ cup of vinegar 3 ½ cups of hot water Put in a spray bottle
Furniture Cleaner	**Washbasin, Bathtub, Tiles**
1/8 cup olive oil 1 tablespoon vinegar 1 tablespoon vodka	½ cup of baking soda 2-3 tablespoons of vinegar Wipe with soft cloth
Wood Floors, Panels	**Stained Mugs**
1 ½ cups of vinegar 1 ½ cups of hot water 20 drops of chosen essential oil	1 teaspoon baking soda 1 teaspoon water Make into paste

TOXINS IN OUR FOODS

Herbicides and pesticides are used in conventional farming to deter pests and increase yields. Chronic exposure to the corn herbicide Atrazine has been linked to mitochondrial dysfunction, leading to weight gain and insulin resistance. This herbicide has also been found in our water systems, and has been linked to obesity. Most of our corn is grown in the Midwest, and there is an overlap of where the herbicide is used and where obesity is prevalent.

Eating Organic Foods

According to the Environmental Workgroup, a nonprofit consumer protection agency, some non-organic produce may be especially contaminated with pesticides. Many of these foods are heavily sprayed with pesticides to the point that workers have to wear gas masks.

2012 Dirty Dozen:

Foods with highest pesticide residues
1. Apples
2. Celery
3. Sweet bell peppers
4. Peaches
5. Strawberries
6. Nectarines
7. Grapes
8. Spinach
9. Lettuce
10. Cucumbers
11. Blueberries
12. Potatoes
**Non-organic green beans and kale also contained a high amount of pesticides

---

2012 Clean Fifteen: Foods with lowest pesticide residues
1) Onions
2) Sweet Corn
3) Pineapples
4) Avocado
5) Cabbage
6) Sweet Peas
7) Asparagus
8) Mangos
9) Eggplant
10) Kiwi
11) Cantaloupe
12) Sweet potatoes
13) Grapefruit
14) Watermelon
15) Mushrooms

Heavy Metals

Heavy metals may also interfere with thyroid function. Mercury fillings in particular have been found to be problematic in those with Hashimoto's. As mercury is a metal that becomes vapor when heated, the heat generated from the friction of chewing causes it to be released into circulation. Removing mercury fillings (by a specialized holistic dentist) is greatly recommended and has been associated with a reduction in TPO antibodies.

Additional sources of mercury have been found in fish. Tuna contains a lot of mercury and should be avoided, while anchovies, salmon, flounder, and whitefish may be enjoyed up to twice per week.

Other metals can also leach into our bodies. Aluminum is the most common and is present in antiperspirants and some cooking pans. Nonstick pans that are scratched are a source of leaks. Stainless steel cookware is recommended instead.

Table 15: Mercury Levels in Fish:

Adapted from americanpregnancy.org/pregnancyhealth/**fishmercury**.htm

Highest Mercury: **AVOID** Eating	High Mercury: Eat no more than three 6-oz servings per month	Lower Mercury: Eat no more than six 6-oz servings per month	Lowest Mercury: Enjoy two 6-oz servings per week
Marlin Orange roughy Tilefish Swordfish Shark Mackerel (king) Tuna (bigeye, ahi)	Sea Bass (Chilean) Bluefish Grouper Mackerel (Spanish, gulf) Tuna (canned, white albacore) Tuna (yellowfin)	Bass (striped, black) Carp Cod (Alaskan) Croaker (White Pacific) Halibut (Pacific and Atlantic) Jacksmelt (silverside) Lobster Mahi-Mahi Monkfish Perch (freshwater) Sablefish Skate Snapper Sea Trout (Weakfish) Tuna (canned, chunk light) Tuna (Skipjack)	Anchovies Butterfish Catfish Clam Crab (domestic) Crawfish/crayfish Croaker Flounder Haddock Hake Herring Mackerel (North Atlantic, chub) Mullet Oysters Perch (ocean) Plaice Salmon Sardines Scallops Shad (American) Shrimp Sole Squid (calamari) Tilapia Trout (freshwater) Whitefish Whiting

BODY'S DETOXIFICATION SYSTEM

We have an innate detoxification system that can help us clear toxins from foods, chemicals, and other exposures. However, when our body can't keep up with elimination of toxins because of compromised digestion, toxins accumulate in our cells and the fluid around the cells (extracellular fluid).

Our bodies' cells take in nutrients and oxygen from the blood, perform their functions, and then give off waste products. The waste products are expelled from the cells into the extracellular matrix where they undergo an exchange with the bloodstream for the nutrients coming in. The blood transports these wastes to the liver to be detoxified and then to the organs of elimination: the intestine, kidneys, lungs and skin, for final disposal. When our organs are burdened with excessive wastes, they show signs of their stress.

Skin: Rashes, pimples, or offensive body odor
Kidneys: Frequent, painful, or urgent urination or dark or offensive-smelling urine
Liver: Gas, diarrhea, and constipation or green, mucous stools, or right-sided chest pain
Lungs: Congestion, coughs, or wheezing

Each person may show different signs of stress, depending on their particular weakness and the toxins to which they are exposed.

Liver

The liver is our main detoxification organ, and proper liver function is necessary to convert T4 to the active T3 hormone. In addition, the liver filters blood, stores glucose for energy, breaks down steroid hormones, and produces/secretes bile, which is necessary for fat

275

digestion. The liver also gets rid of toxins we encounter. Liver function may be impaired in those with Hashimoto's.

The elimination of toxins by the liver is done through a two-step enzymatic process.

Phase I

During Phase I, a family of enzymes known as Cytochrome P450 Enzymes (CYP450) metabolizes fat-soluble toxins into intermediary substances. Substances such as foods, drugs, and toxins undergo various processes such as: oxidation, reduction, hydrolysis, hydration, and dehalogenation in order to prepare them to attach to detoxifying nutrients in Phase II.

These intermediates are often more toxic then the original substances ingested.

The required nutrients in Phase I are B vitamins (B_2, B_3, B_6, B_{12}, folic acid, glutathione, and flavonoids).

Phase II

In Phase II, the intermediaries undergo conjugation, sulfation, glucuronidation, glutathione conjugation, acetylation, amino acid conjugation, and methylation reactions, which detoxify them and make them water soluble so that they can be excreted in stool or urine.

The required nutrients in Phase II are folic acid, magnesium, glutathione, B_5, B_{12}, vitamin C; amino acids methionine, cysteine, glycine, taurine, glutamine and choline

As described in the "Depletions" chapter, due to low HCl levels, gluten intolerance and other absorption issues present in Hashimoto's, the body does not properly absorb nutrients that are required for detoxification pathways.

Additionally, as the body is constantly bombarded with toxins in the form of undigested foods, pesticides, medications, exhaust fumes, etc., this results in a "backlog" or "liver congestion," where the toxins build up, get back into the blood, and/or are stored in our fat.

Drug Metabolism and the Liver

CYP450 enzymes are the primary mode of drug metabolism in our bodies. Some medications can saturate, speed up, or slow down the enzymes, which can lead to adverse drug events and drug-to-drug interactions.

Tylenol® overdose: Tylenol® is a medication commonly used for headaches, pain, and fevers. When taking Tylenol® at normal doses, without any interacting drugs or liver impairment, the liver converts the Tylenol® into a toxic intermediary, which is then quickly bound by glutathione and eliminated. When the total daily dose of Tylenol® exceeds 4 grams per day, the body runs out of glutathione, and the toxic metabolite builds up, leading to liver failure and even death.

N-Acetylcysteine (which converts to glutathione) is given to people who overdose on Tylenol® to help the liver clear the toxic metabolite.

Some medications as well as a substance found in grapefruit can inhibit liver enzymes, and lead to a toxic buildup of medications that require the particular enzymes for metabolism.

Signs that your detoxification system may be impaired include:
- ☐ Digestion, elimination problems
- ☐ Inability to lose or gain weight
- ☐ Allergies, congestion, etc.
- ☐ Skin disorders such as acne
- ☐ Fatigue
- ☐ Anger
- ☐ Depression
- ☐ Irritability
- ☐ Dark circles under eyes
- ☐ Blood sugar imbalances
- ☐ Hormonal imbalances
- ☐ PMS
- ☐ Asthma
- ☐ Frequent infections
- ☐ Joint and muscle pains
- ☐ Insomnia
- ☐ Chemical sensitivities

ACID ALKALINE FOOD BALANCE

Creating a more alkaline environment in the body may help with the detoxification process as well as help alkaline phosphatase function better. While this initially seems contradictory to the previous recommendation of increasing stomach acidity, it is not. Keeping the stomach acidic while the rest of the body alkaline is the key to optimal health, and can be achieved through diet and digestive enzymes.

The alkaline and acidic properties of foods are very confusing, mostly because people use the same terminology to describe the taste of the food, as well as whether our body needs to produce more acid or alkaline enzymes to digest the food.

A food such as a tomato, for example, may be considered an acidic food to those who eat it, but it requires alkaline enzymes to digest it, and thus leaves a net alkaline residue in the body.

In contrast, milk doesn't taste acidic, but requires acidic enzymes to be digested.

Foods that are high in protein but low in potassium are generally going to be acidic. This includes most meats, dairy, some nuts, and cereals/grains that are poor in potassium. Additionally, most processed foods are considered acidic as well.

In contrast, foods rich in potassium but low in protein, such as fruits and vegetables, require an alkaline environment for digestion.

Eating too many animal products and starches without the correct balance from alkaline vegetables and fruit may create a net acidic residue in the body, but will not help make the stomach more acidic. Additionally, taking digestive enzymes to acidify the stomach (which needs to be acidic) will not affect the acid/base ratio of the rest of the body.

Protein based acidic foods are important for building up the body, while the alkaline foods detoxify our bodies. Both types of foods are required for proper health.

A ratio of 20% acidic foods to 80% alkaline foods has been suggested for a proper acid/alkaline balance. As we are all different, this ratio may not be appropriate for everyone and different ratios may be utilized depending on whether our bodies need more building or cleansing.

Not all acidic foods are equal. Some acidic foods, such as organic eggs, meat, and animal fat may be nutritious, while others like refined flour, sugar, and processed vegetable oils are detrimental, and should always be limited. While the nutritious acidic foods are required for proper body function, they should be limited when attempting to detoxify/cleanse the body.

Additionally, not all alkaline foods are equal when attempting to cleanse. Raw fruits and vegetables are more alkaline than their cooked counterparts. Almonds and cashews are two nuts that are generally considered to be more alkaline, but not everyone may be able to tolerate them. Raw fruits, vegetables, herbs, and spices have the most potent detoxifying effects.

Cleansing should be done one to two times per year for a period of one to two weeks, but long-term diets that rely on alkaline foods at the exclusion of nutritious acid foods are not recommended for Hashimoto's.

Acidic Foods	Alkaline Foods
Meat	Fruits
Dairy	Vegetables
Eggs	Greens
Processed foods	Most nuts
Fats	Seeds
Sugar	Beans
Flour	Potatoes
Fried foods	Gluten-free grains

What is a Detoxification Protocol?

Detoxification is a broad term that is used to describe a variety of different methods that can help cleanse the body's internal system and organs.

Detoxification protocols may include nutritional supplementation, herbal medicines, raw vegetarian diets, fasting, juicing, probiotics, hydrotherapy, sauna, colonic irrigation, and exercise.

Detoxification addressed four different types of toxins: heavy metals, chemical toxins, microbial compounds, and byproducts from protein metabolism.

Why Detoxify?

Detoxification protocols cleanse the body of buildup accumulated as a result of our dietary habits, toxic environment, and an overburdened detoxification system. Proponents of detoxification report clearer skin, reduced symptoms of many conditions, improved vitamin and mineral absorption, and improved bowel function.

AUTOIMMUNE DETOX

Detoxification is an important part of re-establishing healthy thyroid function. The liver is our main detoxification organ, but may become "congested," for a lack of a better word, because of all of the toxic substances we are exposed to on a daily basis.

Avoiding alcohol, caffeine, pesticides, and chemicals is a great way to start the detoxification process. However, sometimes additional intervention may be required.

Detox Methods

I researched a variety of detox methods, as I wanted to develop a detox program that fit the needs of those with Hashimoto's.

Fasting is a great way to detox, but may exacerbate adrenal fatigue. Fiber and vegetables that are rich in sulfur also support liver detoxification, as do raw fruits and vegetables. However, I knew that raw fruits and vegetables were not an option for those with very impaired digestion. Additionally, fiber may be very aggravating to many of those with Hashimoto's due to small-intestinal bacterial overgrowth.

Generally, detox diets eliminate animal proteins and rely on nuts and seeds for protein, however, these may also be too difficult to digest for some people with Hashimoto's.

I was looking into all of the products available for liver detoxing, and most of the products on the market are powders that are made into shakes to be taken as replacements for meals.

Most of the products contain rice, soy, or dairy as a source of protein, which may be problematic to people who have Hashimoto's and associated PAIRs and food sensitivities. Additionally, most products contain insoluble fiber, which can be fermented by the pathogenic bacteria and perpetuate autoimmunity.

I scratched my head for months, until someone recommended the movie "Fat, Sick and Nearly Dead." For those who have not seen the movie, it is about a man who is able to put his autoimmune condition (chronic urticaria) in remission by following a sixty-day juice fast.

A juicer machine is used to extract the liquid from fruits and vegetables. The liquid is easy to absorb by the body and only contains vitamins, minerals, and enzymes, as well as some soluble fiber that will bind toxins, while the insoluble fiber is left behind. We get most of the benefits of raw fruits and vegetables without putting the extra stress of digestion on our body, and allow our bodies to rest and regenerate.

Approaches to Detox

- **Vitamins and minerals** that are necessary for proper liver function are used to support the body's internal detoxification pathway.
- **Detoxifying herbs** are thought to bind toxins to help with their breakdown and excretion. Some herbs also work by stimulating the liver's detoxifying ability.
- **Foods and diet:** Clean diets give the body a break from being burdened by toxins from foods, allowing the body to process the backlog of accumulated toxins.
- **Fasting:** In fasting the body breaks down fat for fuel, this is thought to help with eliminated wastes that accumulate in our fat tissues.
- **Hydrotherapy:** Hot water and baths stimulate blood circulation through the liver, helping the liver filter out more toxins. Toxins are also excreted through sweat.
- **Probiotics:** Probiotics help to minimize harmful gut bacteria that make toxins and help preserve the protective intestinal lining allowing for toxic substances to pass through the digestive track for elimination.
- **Sauna:** The heat in saunas stimulates blood circulation and sweating allowing for more effective excretion of toxins.
- **Colonic irrigation:** Flushing the colon with water and herbs is believed to flush out the toxins that accumulate in the lining of the intestinal tract.
- **Toxin binding:** When taken internally, fiber and clay are thought to bind to toxins and heavy metals present in our intestinal tract and aid with their excretion from the body.
- **Exercise:** Exercise helps with detoxification by increasing blood and lymphatic flow throughout the body's filtration system and also helps excrete toxins through sweat.

Adapted from Natural Standard Database

Although the man in the movie transitioned to a vegan diet after the juice fast, we know that vegan, raw diets, and fasting diets are not optimal for those with Hashimoto's. This is because people with Hashimoto's are depleted in many of the nutrients typically obtained from animal sources: (zinc, ferritin iron, selenium, and fatty acids). We also know that animal proteins are the hardest to digest, and are often not digested properly by those with Hashimoto's because of low hydrochloric acid.

Therefore, taking a one to fourteen day break from animal protein and giving the body an opportunity to take a rest from digestion can be very regenerative for the gut and liver. Soups and broths can give the bowels a rest and can help restore the intestinal lining but may not provide all of the required micronutrients that are often found in fresh fruits and vegetables, which are necessary for detoxification.

That's When the Juice and Soup Fast was Born

This fast fits with the Hashimoto's protocol and the Elimination diet, and at the same time helps to address the depletions present due to absorption issues in Hashimoto's.

The fast is started with two to three days of homemade broth mixed to a puree consistency with well-cooked low-residue vegetables that include carrots, zucchini, and pumpkin. The vegetables should be prepared with ample fatty acids such as coconut oil, duck fat, lard, and cod liver oil. A tablespoon of coconut oil is added to each soup.

Juices are introduced after three days for those without diarrhea. In the case of diarrhea, they may need to be pushed out by a few weeks. Juices should be taken preferably on an empty stomach, before the soups. Drinking purified water and herbal teas can be both soothing and relaxing. It is also important to start a probiotic regimen at this time. The juice fast is a low-residue diet, and will likely begin to cause die-off from the bacteria in the small intestine.

After a few days of combining the juice with the soup, the person can transition off the soups into a full juice cleanse, lasting anywhere between one and seven days. Afterwards, the soups are added back in, and we transition back into introducing meats and other more difficult to digest foods. Alternately, smoothies of well-pureed raw vegetables can be used in place of the juices.

Fruit should be limited to low-fructose fruits like granny smith apples, lemons, limes, and tomatoes, and should be used in mixture with vegetable juices. Goitrogenic raw vegetables should be limited.

Some ideas for juicing vegetables include carrots, celery, cucumber, zucchini, and leafy greens. Small amounts of apple may be added to sweeten the juices, but it is important not to use too many fruits due to their high sugar content. Lemons also mix well with juices.

Small amounts of ginger root, onion, or turmeric root may also be added to the juice.

Juice Ideas

Purified water with the juice of one lemon (may add Stevia)

2 stalks of celery, ½ of a green apple, 2 large carrots, ½ inch of ginger root

½ cucumber, 1 tomato, 4 carrots, ½ inch turmeric root

1 bunch or parsley, 1 zucchini, 2 carrots, 1 lemon, 5 leaves and stems of basil, 1 green apple

---

TOXIN BINDERS

Lemon juice

Lemon juice has cleansing properties and helps detoxify the liver. It can be taken in the morning on an empty stomach with a half-cup of purified water or mixed with vegetable juice.

Fiber

Fiber helps bind the toxins and eliminates them through stool. Fiber found in fresh fruit and vegetables such as inulin, FOS, and psyllium husk are healthful fibers that may aid with binding toxins, however, they may be too abrasive for those with increased intestinal permeability and may aggravate small-intestinal bacterial overgrowth.

Bentonite Clay

Bentonite clay also has strong cleansing and absorptive properties when taken internally. It is gentler for those with gastrointestinal issues and has been helpful for people who have irritable bowel syndrome.

The clay is not absorbed by the body or fermented by the intestinal bacteria, and actually attracts and binds toxins such as viruses, parasites, heavy metals, pesticides, and chemicals as it passes through the intestinal tract. The toxin-filled clay is expelled in bowel movements.

In addition to being taken internally, clay can be used in baths and for facials as it helps detoxify the body through the pores of the skin.

The clay should not be taken during pregnancy, and should be spaced out from medications by at least two hours as it is likely to bind the medication as well. Bentonite clay is available in liquid or powder form. The liquid may taste better.

Detox Supplements

The required nutrients for Phase I and II liver detoxification include: B vitamins (B_2, B_3, B_5, B_6, B_{12}), folic acid, glutathione, flavonoids, magnesium, vitamin C, and the amino acids methionine, cysteine, glycine, taurine and glutamine.

N-Acetyl Cysteine

N-Acetyl Cysteine, which turns into glutathione, not only helps reduce TPO antibodies by neutralizing hydrogen peroxide, and helps heal intestinal permeability but also aids with detoxification. Doses of 1.8 grams (1,800 mg) are usually recommended.

Amino Acids

Amino acids are necessary for rebuilding and healing the body. Proteins are our major source of amino acids, however, protein breakdown is burdensome on the body and takes away from healing and cleansing. Pure amino acids require no work on the part of the body and are easily absorbable, however, they taste disgusting. Prolonged juice fasts that exclude proteins may result in protein deficiency, and supplementing with pure amino acids mixed with cranberry juice and Stevia or in supplement form may help support the body in its rebuilding efforts.

Herbs

A variety of herbs has been reported to be helpful with cleansing and many commercial "liver detox support" products may have one or more of the following ingredients, sometimes in combination with the vitamins/supplements listed above.

Table 16: Substances That Support Liver Detox

Artichoke	Barberry	Boldo	Fringetree
Dandelion	Alfalfa	Beet	Lecithin
Milk Thistle	Licorice	Capsicum	Cellulose
Schisandra	Turmeric	Phosphatidylcholine	

Chlorella/Spirulina

Chlorella and spirulina are sometimes recommended as detox supplements, but they may have some immune stimulating properties that can induce or exacerbate autoimmune conditions, through the upregulation of TNF-A (the Th-1 branch). This same reaction has also been reported with echinacea. There have been a few cases of new onset autoimmune conditions following the use of these supplements, therefore, I don't recommend them.

Activities to Support Detox

In addition to diet and supplements, a variety of activities may also be helpful with the detox process, including Epsom salt baths, enemas, colon cleansing, massage therapy, and oil pulling.

Skin

The skin is a major elimination organ for toxins as well. Sweating especially helps to eliminate toxins. Low production of sweat is a symptom of hypothyroidism (although not one many people complain about). As people with hypothyroidism usually have a lower body temperature, they often need to make themselves sweat. This can be done by exercise, the use of saunas, hot baths or my favorite, hot yoga. Additionally, brushing the skin may be helpful with eliminating toxins.

Colon

Elimination of toxins is also done through the gastrointestinal tract. In some cases, when we are detoxifying, the toxins may not clear out efficiently from our bowel, and we may become backed up. Enemas and colon cleanses may be helpful with elimination of toxins, especially for those who are more on the constipated side.

Cleansing the colon supports detoxification and stimulates the liver to dump bile. It is especially important for those who are not having regular bowel movements.

The use of enemas as well as colonics may be helpful with increasing waste elimination and reducing the unpleasant symptoms associated with detoxing that occur because the body is not clearing toxins quickly enough.

Enemas can be done at home, while colonics are administered by specially trained colon hydrotherapists who use sterilized equipment to introduce fluid into the colon to irrigate it.

Lymphatic System

The lymph system is also responsible for transporting toxins around our body and facilitating their elimination. Increasing lymphatic flow consists of lifestyle modifications that almost everyone enjoys. It can be done through bouncing on a trampoline (or mini-trampoline), massages, and inversion exercises such as my favorite yoga pose, the shoulder-stand. Woo hoo!

Massage Therapy

Massage therapy helps with tissue cleansing and is a wonderful relaxing detoxification tool. Massage induces the release of toxins from the tissues and facilitates their elimination. It turns the extracellular matrix from a jelly-like substance into a more liquid state, allowing it to be eliminated better.

Remember to drink plenty of pure water before and after a massage to further enhance your elimination and to replenish your body's supply of water.

HALOGEN DETOX

Halogens are more likely to accumulate in the case of iodine deficiency. However, we know that iodine itself also acts as a trigger for Hashimoto's, and can perpetuate the autoimmune attack.

It is important to reduce iodine intake while we work to eliminate thyroid antibodies. Once the antibodies have been eliminated, we will start introducing iodine back in, in order to facilitate thyroid hormone production.

Some physicians report that "halogen detox" may occur when reintroducing iodine, which presents as acne, palpitations, and other detox symptoms.

Once TPO is no longer positive, we can start supplementing with iodide, but very, very gradually.

Chapter Summary

- ✓ Toxins are found in foods and personal products.
- ✓ Mercury, and halogens like fluoride, bromide, and chloride have been associated with Hashimoto's and thyroid dysfunction.
- ✓ The liver is our main detoxification organ.
- ✓ Cleansing allows the body to rest and get rid of toxins.

PART III: HOW TO HEAL

"Every day in every way, I am getting better and better."- Émile Coué

17: GETTING BETTER

One thing to remember about overcoming Hashimoto's is that it takes many years to develop the perfect storm of Hashimoto's Thyroiditis. Thus, healing won't happen overnight.

Healing Hashimoto's is a marathon, not a sprint, and the life changes you make will gradually lead to a healthier, more balanced you.

It is important to keep a positive outlook and avoid negative feelings, our negative emotions wreak havoc on gut and adrenal function, two of the main promoters of autoimmunity!

In the beginning, we discussed the three approaches to Hashimoto's...eliminating triggers, restoring depletions and restoring gut function.

Eliminating triggers: Triggers will take quite some time to discover and eliminate. A trigger for one person may not be a trigger for another.

This book is based on current research, but may be missing other triggers and factors that contribute to Hashimoto's. Eliminating triggers like infections, iodine, gluten, food intolerances, fluoride, and other toxins may take a few days to a few months.

Depletions: Building up your levels of vitamins and nutrients may take a few months to a year.

Gut function: Bacterial overgrowth, candida overgrowth, gut dysbiosis, and adrenal dysfunction may take six months to two years to stabilize.

In the meantime, thyroid hormone supplementation, immune modulation, and throwing the immune system a decoy are options available to you to prevent further thyroid damage.

So now you have all of this information, and your head is probably spinning. How can you use all of this information to get better? I recommend starting with putting together your health timeline. This will help you identify your potential triggers.

Next, you can either write out a problem list of all of the things you are undergoing, or use the journals, quizzes, and tracking tools at www.thyroidrootcause.org/guide to track your progress.

This will help you determine which types of tests and interventions may be helpful to implement.

The approach to healing is fourfold: diet, supplements, lifestyle changes, and medications, when indicated.

You Are Unique

Bio-individuality is a concept that everyone is biologically unique, or to put it plainly, everyone is different. Thus it is possible that some strategies that worked for one person may make another person worse. It is important to pay careful attention and to keep track of your own progress in your healing journey.

How Will You Know a Change is an Improvement?

Journaling, testing, and keeping track of your symptoms will help you determine if your healing journey is heading in the right direction.

Balancing Measures

As you may notice, many of the supplements that can be helpful for Adrenals—astragalus, DHEA, licorice root, and the thyroid (selenium, glutathione, algae) may actually increase the Th-1 branch, perpetuating immune imbalance.

Perhaps an immune imbalance depletes these nutrients, causing thyroid and adrenal dysfunction, and once the nutrients are depleted the overactive branch gets burned out. By supporting the thyroid and adrenals we end up inadvertently supporting the overactive arm as well.

Candida and fungal infections shift the immune system towards producing more Th-2 cells. Viruses and Gram-negative bacteria produce more Th-1 cells. Getting rid of a candida or parasitic infection may shift the immune system to Th-1 if there is a chronic viral infection or Gram-negative bacteria present.

It is important to keep this balance in mind while attempting to restore one part of the system, not to worsen another part. If antibodies worsen or new symptoms develop suggestive of a Th-1 dominance, it may be helpful to start some Th-2 stimulating substances to help restore the balance.

Autoimmune Flare, Intolerance, or Healing Crisis?

A die-off reaction, also known as a Jarisch-Herxheimer reaction, or sometimes just Herxheimer or "Herx," is a reaction that occurs when in their death, the detrimental bacteria release toxins at a quicker rate than the body can clear them.

This type of reaction can occur with changes in diet, such as eliminating sugars, starches, or fiber,(which is sometimes referred to as starving the pathogenic bacteria); and with increasing fermented foods containing beneficial bacteria that displace the pathogenic bacteria through competition. It can also occur after starting probiotics, digestive enzymes, and antibiotics.

Symptoms of die-off may include: lethargy, difficulty concentrating, craving sweets, diarrhea, rash, irritability, gas, bloating, headache, nausea, vomiting, increased autoimmune symptoms, and congestion.

These symptoms usually resolve within a few days but have been reported to last for many weeks in some cases. When the symptoms occur in response to the above-mentioned interventions, they are generally associated with a healing crisis. Pushing through, or doing colon cleansing, skin brushing, detox baths, and taking Anatabine and curcumin may be helpful in managing these symptoms.

Intolerances are associated with some of the same symptoms, however, they occur in the absence of these interventions and in response to foods. When these symptoms occur after ingesting any of the substances mentioned in the "Intolerance" chapter, they should be especially suspect.

An autoimmune flare can result when the wrong type of immune balancing intervention is used, or when balance is restored in one part of the system but not another. Please see the Naranjo Causality Scale in the "Supplements" chapter for a guide on how to determine the likely intervention that is causing an adverse event. The suspected interventions should be stopped. Autoimmune flares should be treated with acupuncture or with counterbalancing supplements.

Challenges of Lifestyle Interventions

Lifestyle interventions for Hashimoto's and autoimmune conditions are still in their infancy. This research is not yet well known and accepted by the traditional medical system or our society in general.

Friends and family and even your physicians may be skeptical when you tell them that you are no longer going to follow the Standard American Diet in an effort to overcome your autoimmune condition. You may be overwhelmed by the notion of changing so many routines and cutting out your favorite foods.

I know that lifestyle changes are challenging. It is certainly much easier to take a pill on a daily basis rather than follow diets, reduce stress and exercise. However, please consider the following statistic…

Fifty million people in the United States have an autoimmune condition. That is a whopping 20% of our population!

Every system is perfectly designed to get the results it gets.

Thus our society, medical system and diet are perfectly designed to produce 50 million people with autoimmunity. It's up to you to decide if you want to be like everyone else and get the same results they get, or try a different approach to your health.

Getting help

Unfortunately most traditionally trained medical professionals believe that Synthroid® and the TSH are all there is to managing Hashimoto's. While these professionals can get you on the right track with the medication component of the condition, they may not be very helpful with lifestyle interventions such as diet and supplements.

Nonetheless, you should see your physician on a quarterly basis to have your thyroid medication and function monitored. The physicians will help you determine if your thyroid has recovered to the point of being able to reduce the thyroid medication.

In addition, I would recommend working with a professional who is well versed in nutrition and functional medicine.

You should consider making one or more of the following professionals as part of your health care team:

- Functional medicine practitioners- are trained in treating the body as whole, integrating lifestyle interventions

- Chiropractors-chiropractors have an exceptional understanding of human physiology and many pursue advanced education in nutrition

- Naturopaths- naturopaths focus on restoring the body's innate ability to heal often through nutritional means

- Compounding or Integrative Pharmacists- many of these pharmacists pursue advanced nutrition training especially in the realms of hormone balancing and nutritional healing

- Acupuncturists-acupuncture is an ancient healing art that can help to balance the immune system

- Nutritionists/Diet Coaches-holistic nutrition professionals can help design a healing diet that is appropriate for your needs

If you are unable to find a practitioner in your area, I also provide phone consultations for a limited number of clients.

Healing Hashimoto's Summary

In addition to appropriate diagnosis and proper medication management, my approach for overcoming Hashimoto's is as follows:

First, we remove the things that may be irritating your thyroid and causing it to send out a stress signal. Iodine, fluoride, and toxins can cause thyroid inflammation as a result of oxidative damage, causing the thyroid to send out a stress response, which becomes picked up by the immune system.

Gluten and food intolerances promote intestinal permeability, making our immune system unable to recognize our own cells. Food that is poorly digested feeds the bad bacteria, making them stronger.

Stress weakens the thyroid through its actions on the adrenals, AND can help the negative bacteria proliferate. We strengthen the adrenals by balancing the blood sugar and reducing stress. The adrenals also respond well to adaptogens.

Second, we repair the intestinal permeability through a leaky gut diet, broths, and glutamine. Protomorphogens are used as a decoy for thyroid and adrenal glands, and help rebuild the organs.

Third, we replace the depletions that are present to help the body strengthen and jump back on a cycle of wellness. This includes thyroid hormone!

Fourth, we reinoculate, giving the body enough beneficial bacteria to displace the pathogenic bacteria. Probiotics and raw lacto-fermented foods are used.

Lastly, we rebalance our immune system and detoxification capabilities.

The immune system can be balanced with anatabine and curcumin supplements. The green juices, smoothies and vegetables are used to make the body more alkaline to help optimize the function of alkaline phosphatase enzyme so it can detoxify endotoxin from pathogenic bacteria more efficiently.

The complete approach to healing Hashimoto's can be summarized through the Five R's of Healing an approach used by Functional Medicine Practitioners that I have tailored for Hashimoto's patients.

The Five R's of Healing Hashimoto's

Remove
- Iodine
- Infections
- Fluoride
- Toxins
- Difficult to digest food
- Food intolerances
- Stress

Repair
- Healing diet
- Protomorphogens
- Broths
- Glutamine

Replace
- B_{12}
- Zinc
- Selenium
- Ferritin
- Other vitamin and mineral depletions
- Thyroid hormone
- Digestive enzymes

Reinoculate
- Probiotics
- Fermented Foods

Rebalance
- Adrenal adaptogens
- Anatabine/Curcumin/Omega-3's
- Green juices, smoothies, vegetables

"He who takes medicine and neglects to diet wastes the skill of his doctors."-Chinese Proverb

18: Diet for Hashimoto's

What is the right diet to heal Hashimoto's?

This question is very complicated, and unfortunately, nutrition is the only science where multiple answers can be both correct and wrong. In other words, there is more than one way to skin a cat, and one man's medicine may be another man's poison.

As we know, the three factors for thyroid autoimmunity are 1) genes 2) trigger(s) 3) intestinal permeability. While we can't change genes, we can change their expression by removing triggers and correcting intestinal permeability. For some, it may be as easy as removing excess iodine intake, and cutting out gluten (a major cause of increased intestinal permeability).

For others, it may require a significant amount of lifestyle change, including diets and interventions aimed at removing parasitic, fungal, bacterial, and viral infections, environmental triggers, coupled with removal of offending foods, balancing blood sugar as well as the addition of healing foods and stress reduction.

We are all different, and although we may have the same condition, different interventions may be required for each of us to heal.

Multiple diets have been reported to reverse Hashimoto's and/or other autoimmune conditions, including a gluten-free diet, iodine-free diet, Feingold Diet, Specific Carbohydrate Diet, GAPS Diet, The Paleo Diet, Autoimmune Paleo Diet, soy-free diet, dairy-free diet, low-FODMAPs Diet, the Body Ecology Diet, and elemental diet.

The connecting thread behind these diverse diets, is that they all remove various reactive foods. Most of the diets include animal proteins, are more nutrient dense than the Standard American Diet, and remove processed foods. Many of the diets recommend healing foods like fermented foods or gelatins.

While vegan and vegetarian diets have been reported to be extremely helpful with autoimmune and chronic conditions, I have not been able to find reports of people recovering from Hashimoto's by following a vegan diet. Even devout vegans who are nutritionally conscious still struggle with low body temperatures, hypothyroidism and Hashimoto's.

Additionally, many former vegans have reported improved symptoms of Hashimoto's following transitioning to a Paleo diet. Based on this, I believe that animal proteins must play an important role in building back the health of people with Hashimoto's.

That said, while meats and fats are important for healing, eating them exclusively will produce an acidic environment in the body; hindering healing, and thus the diet should be balanced with plenty of nutrient rich vegetables (suggested ratio may be 20% meat/80% veggie).

Additionally, vegan and raw vegan diets can be extremely helpful for cleansing and detoxifying, especially for those with persistent protein digestion issues. A vegan diet can be followed for a few days to a few weeks and may help the body detoxify. B_{12} and iron or ferritin supplements should be utilized at this time to prevent deficiency.

Another approach may be to follow a "semi-vegan" diet or the "Morning Vegan" approach, where one eats primarily vegan foods (nuts, seeds, veggies) for breakfast and lunch but consumes a meat based meal for dinner.

<u>Which of these is right for me?</u>

While it's hard to predict who will do well with which approach, generally those with a history of gastrointestinal issues (IBS, GERD, stomachaches, food intolerances), antibiotic, oral contraceptive use, and high-carbohydrate diets will require more time and lifestyle changes for healing.

Variables such as being underweight/normal weight, younger age at onset of symptoms (<30 y/o) may also mean that more comprehensive and complex approaches must be followed.

THE PERFECT DIET?

Intestinal permeability may be caused by small-intestinal bacterial overgrowth, dysbiosis, Candida, parasites or reactions to foods, or in many cases, a vicious cycle of all of the above.

Many individualized factors should be taken into account when designing a diet for overcoming Hashimoto's, such as individual food reactions, the compositions of one's intestinal flora, the presence of blood sugar abnormalities, depletions, the presence of infections, and the person's ability to digest and absorb nutrients from foods.

Working with a nutritionist or coach specially trained in thyroid/autoimmune diets may be extremely helpful in developing an individualized healing diet.

The principles of a healing dietary protocol are as follows.
1) The dietary protocol should take the person's individuality into account.
2) The dietary protocol should remove triggering foods.
3) The dietary protocol should add healing foods.
4) The dietary protocol should replenish nutrients.

The following diets are meant to be utilized for healing, but may not be necessarily followed indefinitely. For some, components of otherwise healthful diets such as fruit and fiber might need to be temporarily limited to help with healing.

Considerations for Individualizing the Dietary Approach

The limitation of the FODMAPs and Paleo diets is that they do not take into account the individuality of each person. One person may do just fine with dairy, while another may react terribly to it. These diets should thus be used as a guide to develop a personalized approach for overcoming an autoimmune thyroid disorder.

The SCD, GAPS and Body Ecology diets are programs that focus on healing and sealing the intestinal lining, by first removing offending agents, and then adding back nutritious foods and probiotics, allowing our digestion to catch up.

The programs start with an Introduction Phase. Think of the introduction phase as a "baby food phase," as these types of "introduction" diets are also fed to babies, who have increased intestinal permeability.

The diets start with broths, soups, and purees that are very easy to digest. They advance to well-cooked meats and vegetables, cooked fruits, fruit juices, and eventually raw fruits and vegetables, introducing one new thing every four days or so. The GAPS diet starts off as "low-residue diets," low in indigestible fiber to starve the pathogenic bacteria.

Even with the use of diet and probiotics, the changes in bacterial flora happen very gradually, it may take up to two years for the beneficial bacteria to replace the pathogenic bacteria. The GAPS and

SCD diets need to be continued for one year after the last symptoms until new foods are introduced.

The ability to digest and assimilate nutrients from foods needs to be considered. Some people may require digestive enzymes.

In advanced cases the bacterial flora may be so affected that even fiber in the diet will need to be discontinued for a short time period as it feeds the pathogenic bacterial flora (FODMAPs, Low-Residue, GAPS approach, Elemental Diet).

Small-intestinal bacterial overgrowth (SIBO) may be a cause of a shifted autoimmune response and responsible for Hashimoto's and food intolerances.

The GAPS Diet, SCD Diet, Elemental Diet, FODMAPs Diet, Body Ecology Diet and the new trendy Paleo Diet are examples of diets that can be helpful for overcoming small intestinal bacterial overgrowth, by "starving" out the pathogens and reintroducing beneficial bacteria. Fiber and fruit both can contribute to small intestinal bacterial overgrowth and may also need to be limited.

It is likely that the leaky gut has led to the development of IgG/IgA intolerances to multiple foods. A "baby food" diet may need to be introduced to help prevent further irritation of the intestinal tight junctions in conjunction with healing foods and supplements. In this case, the person will start eating the foods that are easiest to digest, progressing to those that are harder to digest. In the meantime, supplementation with vitamins and minerals is also recommended, as the body is likely not absorbing them. (Elimination/Introduction diet).

Those with protein malabsorption/low stomach acid may benefit from a temporary break from proteins, (animal proteins are the hardest to digest) such as in a juice cleanse, elemental diet or other type of cleanse. Digestive enzymes should also be used with all protein foods.

An overview of the most helpful dietary approaches is listed as follows, starting with the diets requiring the most lifestyle changes, to the diets requiring the fewest lifestyle changes.

Elemental Diet

An elemental diet is a liquid diet that is free of non-digestible substances such as fiber, and contains most of the essential nutrients in a state that requires little to no digestion and results in complete absorption.

The elemental diet is a low-residue diet that is composed of free amino acids and fat in liquid form. Amino acids, glucose, fat and vitamin/mineral supplements are utilized instead of food.

The elemental diet has been traditionally used for rehabilitation of severely malnourished individuals, bowel inflammation, and diarrhea.

The elemental diet results in reduced secretion of pancreatic and gastric juices, giving the stomach and pancreas a rest from activity and allowing for healing and reduction of inflammation to take place. As the diet has very little residue, it results in slower movement of the GI tract, which speeds up healing.

Additionally, free form amino acids allow for the body's own protein to be spared; helping the rest of the body to heal quicker.

An elemental diet may be extremely beneficial in kick starting the process of the thyroid-healing diet. This diet causes a shift in bacterial flora within one to two weeks. This diet requires no digestion on our part, and is an extremely low-residue diet that does not provide any food to the pathogenic bacteria, starving them!

Clinical trials have shown that this diet is effective in reducing SIBO within two weeks in people with IBS, resulting in a great improvement of symptoms.

The limitations of the diet are that amino acids are very expensive to buy, and taste pretty disgusting if not properly prepared. People report feeling nauseated after drinking the solution, and aspiration has resulted when people would lie down too quickly following ingestion.

The formulas that are commercially available (Vivanox®), contain a lot of artificial ingredients that people with Hashimoto's may not tolerate, and contain a lot of carbohydrates that can cause high blood sugars and be detrimental to adrenal function. Additionally, many of the elemental formulas have added iodine.

Some critics of the elemental diets also noticed that symptoms sometimes return after a period of time ranging from months to years. I think this is likely because people go back to their junk food diets too soon. However, if an elemental diet was followed by a grain-free FODMAPS diet, SCD Diet, or similar diet, this could result in permanent remission.

A homemade elemental diet is available at www.thyroidrootcause.org/guide. Note: an elemental diet requires the purchase of very expensive amino acids, and can be quite pricey.

MONOSACCHARIDE DIETS

Monosaccharide diets have a well established track record for healing digestive issues through the exclusion of disaccharide and polysaccharide carbohydrates for a prolonged period of time.

Carbohydrates are sugar molecules and are classified by the number of molecules of sugar that are bound together. Monosaccharides consist of one single sugar molecule and are readily absorbed by the small intestine to provide nutrition for the body. Disaccharides have two sugar molecules bound together, while polysaccharides have multiple sugar molecules bound together.

Polysaccharides and disaccharides are too big to be absorbed by the small intestine, and need to be broken down into monosaccharaides in order to be absorbed into the body.

Carbohydrate Types

Monosaccharide- single sugar molecules
- Glucose
- Fructose
- Galactose
- Found in Fruit, vegetables, honey
- Do not require further breaking down by brush border enzymes to be absorbed

Disaccharides-two sugar molecules bound together
- Lactose
- Sucrose
- Maltose
- Isomaltose
- Found in dairy (lactose) and table sugar (sucrose), from splitting polysaccharides (maltose and isomaltose)

- Need to be spilt by brush border enzymes to be absorbed

Polysaccharides-multiple sugar molecules bound together
- Amylose
- Amylopectin
- Found in potato, rice, wheat and corn
- Need to be spilt by brush border enzymes to be absorbed

Specific Carbohydrate Diet (SCD)

The oldest and most well know monosaccharide diet is the Specific Carbohydrate Diet. This diet was originally designed in the 1920s by a physician named Sydney Haas. This diet was used for overcoming celiac disease, but fell out of favor once gluten was identified as a trigger. The diet re-emerged after Elaine Gottschall, MS, a biochemist and mother of a child who was helped by this diet published a book, "Breaking the Vicious Cycle."

Gottschall proposed adapting a "Specific Carbohydrate Diet" (SCD), a diet that removes starchy carbohydrates like those found in beans, potatoes, and most grains.

People with digestive difficulties have a compromised gut flora. The theory of the diet is that under normal conditions, sucrose and other multiple sugar molecules are broken down by brush border enzymes into the single sugars glucose and fructose, but this does not happen when the flora is compromised. Instead, the villi are so damaged that the molecules do not get broken down. As the body can only absorb single sugars, the molecule is not absorbed and becomes food for the pathogenic gut flora, resulting in gas, toxicity, and more pathogenic bacteria, thus creating a "vicious cycle," as the title of the book proposes.

The SCD excludes polysaccharides/disaccharides (starches) for about a year, and recommends the use of homemade lactose-free yogurt. After being on this diet for at least one year, the villi will regenerate and the person will regain digestive function and eventually be able to tolerate the foods forbidden on the diet.

The diet is kicked-off with an introduction diet that starts with easy to digest foods progressing to more difficult textures with time.

SCD Legal Foods: meat, nuts, most vegetables, fermented foods, seeds, eggs, properly soaked beans, most fruit.

SCD Illegal Foods: sugar, starches, cornstarch, baking powder, chocolate, pectin, potato, maple syrup, molasses, rice, wheat, and all grains (corn, rice, etc.)

Full list of SCD Legal/Illegal foods can be viewed on the website www.breakingtheviciouscycle.info.

The SCD is purported to be effective for people with IBS, Crohn's, celiac disease as well as other digestive issues. Additionally, a modified version of the diet has been adapted to treat behavioral disorders and autoimmune conditions, and is known as the GAPS (Gut and Psychology Syndrome) diet.

GAPS Diet

The Gut and Psychology Syndrome (GAPS) diet by Dr. Natasha Campbell-McBride evolved from the Specific Carbohydrate Diet. Dr. Campbell-McBride modified the diet to help her own son.

The GAPS diet starts with a Healing Phase, which focuses on "healing and sealing" the intestinal lining by removing all irritating foods and providing building blocks for cell repair including amino acids, minerals, fats and fat-soluble vitamins. Fermented foods and probiotics are also started at a low dose and increased over the course of the dietary program.

The healing phase includes homemade broths, soups, animal fat, well-cooked meats, and pureed well-cooked vegetables (zucchini, carrots, pumpkin), while difficult to digest foods such as grains, dairy, fiber, beans, raw fruits and vegetables, and nuts are removed.

The healing phase is continued until all gastrointestinal symptoms have resolved. Although Dr. Campbell-McBride does not provide a specific guideline for how long to follow this phase, as individual results may vary, a good period to allow the healing of the intestines may be two to six weeks.

Following this Healing Phase, foods are gradually added back in during an Introduction Phase, starting with foods that are the easiest to digest. Dr. Campbell-McBride reports that the healing time may vary, and that some people need to stay in the introduction phase for as long as seven months until they are able to tolerate all of the foods on the full GAPS diet. The full GAPS diet, which is very similar to the Paleo and SCD diets, is continued for one to two years before introducing other foods.

Dr. Campbell-McBride reports that skipping the healing phase, as well as introducing foods to soon, may result in difficulty healing and continued food reactions.

Healing phase:
- Stews, soups, fermented foods, bone broth, gelatin
- Meats: all organic (preferred) well-cooked meats allowed
- Vegetables: only low-fiber, well-cooked, pureed

Introduction Diet:
Gradual introduction of foods, starting with the easiest to digest.
1. Well cooked vegetables & meats with soft consistency
2. Soft vegetables/fruit such as avocados, bananas
3. Softly cooked eggs
4. Nut breads
5. Nut butters, soaked nuts
6. Raw fruit, vegetables

Paleo Diet

The full SCD diet and GAPS diets are very similar to the popular Paleo diet that has been gaining attention in mainstream American culture. The theory behind the whole-food, low-carbohydrate Paleo diet is that the digestive systems of humans had not had a chance to adapt to agriculture, yet alone processed foods.

The Paleo diet consists of foods thought to be eaten in the Paleolithic Era by hunter-gatherer tribes, and includes nuts, seeds, meats, eggs, vegetables, and fruit. The diet excludes all processed foods as well as grains. Eggs, dairy, and sweet potatoes are controversial in the Paleo community.

Included: Meat, eggs, nuts, seeds, vegetables, fruit

One can find many delicious recipes that are "Paleo," and a Paleo cookbook is even available at Costco! However, most people need to gradually introduce many of the healthful Paleo foods like in the GAPS diet or SCD diet, rather than go directly into the full diet. The Paleo diet, rich in fiber, can be too difficult to digest for many people with Hashimoto's.

Thus, some call Paleo the "big brother" of SCD.

Autoimmune Gut Repair Diet

Dr. Kharrazian, the author of "Why am I still Having Thyroid Symptoms, When my Lab Tests are Normal?" has recommended a diet similar to the SCD or GAPS diets for healing Hashimoto's.

On his website http://thyroidbook.com/blog/autoimmune-gut-repair-diet/ he recommends an Autoimmune Gut Repair Diet that should be followed for one to sixty days, followed by reintroduction of foods. The diet consists of the following guidelines:

Foods Included
- Most organic vegetables
- Fermented foods
- Most organic meats
- Low-glycemic organic fruits
- Coconut
- Noodles: Brown shirataki yam noodles
- Herbs and Spices

Foods Avoided
- Gluten
- Dairy
- Eggs
- Soy
- Fungi (mushrooms)
- Alcohol
- Beans and legumes
- Nightshades
- Sugars (including honey and agave)
- Canned foods, processed foods, coffee
- High glycemic index foods
- Grains (including buckwheat and rice)
- Nuts and seeds

PATHOGEN TARGETED DIETS

FODMAPs

The FODMAPs approach is a dietary intervention gaining attention among dietitians and the mainstream medical community for its potential efficacy in irritable bowel syndrome (IBS). FODMAPs is an acronym for Fermentable, Oligo-, Di- and Mono-saccharides and Polyols, used to describe the types of carbohydrates that may be fermentable by gut bacteria.

IBS is associated with microflora alterations and malabsorption, and FODMAPs will only induce symptoms in patients to the degree they malabsorb them. Not all FODMAPs will be symptom triggers for all patients. Only those that are malabsorbed are likely to play a role.

FODMAPs found in onions, beans, and garlic are always malabsorbed and will cause gas production in all individuals, even healthy ones. However, people with pathogenic bacteria will have additional symptoms due to the toxic byproducts produced.

Reducing the intake of FODMAPs has been a proposed approach that improves IBS symptoms in about 75% of those who follow this diet.

IBS has been linked to an abnormal gut flora, and the food that we eat can cause a multiplication of the flora. FODMAPs attempts to starve the pathogenic flora by avoiding foods fermented by pathogens. Antibiotics as well as elemental diets are also used for eliminating pathogenic flora.

FODMAPs is different from the SCD, and includes potatoes, gluten-free grains and sugar. It excludes some fruit that contain an excess of

Table 17: FODMAPs Eliminates

FRUCTOSE	LACTOSE	FRUCTANS	GALACTANS	POLYOLS
Apples	Milk	Artichokes	Beans	Apple
Mango	Ice cream	Asparagus	Chickpeas	Apricot
Pear	Yogurt	Beetroot	Kidney	Avocado
Fruit in	Cheese	Broccoli	beans	Blackberry
Juice		Brussels	Lentils	Cherry
Watermelon		sprouts	Soybeans	Peach
Fructose		Cabbage		Pear
HFCS		Eggplant		Plum
Dried fruit		Fennel		Prune
Fruit juice		Garlic		Watermelon
Honey		Leek		Cauliflower
Corn syrup		Okra		Green bell
		Onions		pepper
		Wheat		Mushroom
		Breads		Corn
		Cookies		Sorbitol
		Pasta		Mannitol
		Chicory		Xylitol
		Inulin		

fructose and polyols), fruit juices, honey, some vegetables (avocados, eggplant, onion, etc. due to their fructan content, as well as mushrooms. More information on this type of approach can be found at http://www.ibsgroup.org/brochures/fodmap-intolerances.pdf.

The FODMAPs diet allows some fruits, but it is not recommended to eat too many of them. Bananas, blueberries, boysenberries, cranberries, grapes, grapefruit, honeydew melon, kiwi, lemon, lime, orange, raspberry, and strawberries are allowed.

Vegetables included on FODMAPs are carrots, celery, endive, ginger, green beans, lettuce, olives, parsnips, potato, pumpkin, red bell pepper, spinach, squash, sweet potatoes, tomato, turnip, zucchini, as well as most herbs.

Gluten-free cereals and grains such as rice, oats, polenta, quinoa, psyllium, sorghum, tapioca, and arrowroot are allowed. Most dairy products are not allowed, unless they are lactose-free. Sweeteners such as sugar and maple syrup are allowed, but not in large quantities.

Candida Diet

Candida diet are gluten-, dairy-, sugar-free and low-fructose diets aimed at overcoming the overgrowth of the opportunistic fungus Candida albicans. This fungus may be present in the bodies of those with Hashimoto's.

While modern medicine may find systemic Candida infections controversial, there is some evidence that the opportunistic fungus Candida may be overflowing in some people's guts, especially those who are immune compromised.

Body Ecology Diet

The Body Ecology Diet is a specific type of immune balancing anti-candida diet that may be especially helpful for those with Hashimoto's.

While the GAPS and SCD Diets are grain free and include liberal amounts of nuts, fruit and fruit juices, the Body Ecology Diet includes some well soaked easy to digest grains and limits fruit and nuts to help starve off the pathogenic yeast and bacteria. Additionally, the Body Ecology Diet focuses on foods that create an alkaline environment, allowing alkaline phosphatase to work better to detoxify gram-negative bacteria. Personally, this diet has been extremely helpful in my journey.

Low Fructose Diet

According to researchers from the University of California, San Francisco in the article "The Toxic Truth about Sugar," published in the February 1, 2012 issue of the journal Nature, sugar should be considered a controlled substance just like alcohol and tobacco.

The authors go even further and suggest that sugary foods should be taxed, and sales for kids under 17 years old should be restricted. All of these precautions should be done to make sugar less available, and to encourage other healthful food choices.

Authors Lusting, Schmidt, and Brinds stated that sugar is not just "empty calories" as some claim, but that an excess of sugar is responsible for many diseases in our society. In the last 50 years sugar intake tripled and it is responsible for the global pandemic of obesity, altered metabolism, and high blood pressure. Sugar contributes to an increased death rate from diabetes, heart disease, myocardial infarction, high blood pressure, dyslipidemia, obesity, and cancer. Sugar promotes inflammation and depletes nutrients.

Research has shown that sugar can activate reward pathways in brain like alcohol, morphine, or heroin do.

I can personally attest that I experienced withdrawal symptoms of headaches, irritability, and lethargy for about two weeks after kicking my sugar habit "cold turkey."

According to the American Heart Association, the average American adult consumes 22 teaspoons of sugar daily, while the average teenager consumes 34 teaspoons on a daily basis.

According to the U.S. Department of Agriculture, the average American consumes 156 pounds of sugar per year.

While sugars occur in natural foods like fruits and grains, most of the sugars consumed in the U.S. come from processed foods.

Metabolism of Sugar

The study conducted by nutrition researcher and principal investigator Peter J. Havel, PhD., of the University of California at Davis, showed that fructose and glucose are metabolized in a different way by the body.

Table sugar, or sucrose, is a disaccharide and contains 50% of glucose and 50% fructose. While high-fructose corn syrup is also a disaccharide, and is used in a variety of foods from soft drinks to cereals. It contains 55% of fructose and 45% of glucose.

Glucose is a simple sugar (monosaccharide), and is a product of photosynthesis and the primary source of energy in every cell of our body. Only 20% of glucose is metabolized in liver, while 80% is used by other organs. Excess glucose is converted into glycogen and stored in the liver or muscle, to be covered into glucose when the body needs energy.

When the glucose level increases in blood, insulin is released from the pancreas and helps glucose get into each cell to be used as energy.

Fructose

Fructose is another monosaccharide, and its natural sources are fruits, vegetables, sugar cane, and honey. It can exist in foods as a free fructose or combined with glucose as sucrose. One hundred percent of fructose is metabolized in the liver.

According to Dr. Lusting, fructose is a "chronic, dose dependent liver toxin" and in contrast to glucose, extra fructose is stored as fat when we eat it too much of it. Researchers claim that excess fructose consumption can lead to liver toxicity similar to the kind seen with alcoholic liver disease.

In one study, obese men and women who drank either glucose- or fructose-sweetened beverages as 25% of their calories were followed over a period of ten weeks. Both groups gained weight during the trial but the fat distribution was different. Those in the fructose group added fat in the belly, while the glucose group gained fat under the skin (subcutaneous).

Belly fat has been linked to a high risk of heart disease and diabetes. Besides that, the fructose group had higher cholesterol and LDL "bad cholesterol," and more often had insulin resistance in comparison to the glucose group.

Many Hashimoto's patients have greatly benefitted from limiting fructose and implementing a low carbohydrate or no carbohydrate diet. Excess fructose can be taxing on the liver, feed pathogenic bacteria and yeasts and drive up blood sugar.

As fruit are generally not restricted in the SCD and GAPS Diet, I continued eating liberal amounts of fruit after starting the diet and hit a plateau with my healing progress. As Proteus bacteria ferment fructose, I was essentially providing them ample food despite cutting out so many things and being ultra strict on the SCD. Limiting fructose was a major breakthrough for me and helped me overcome blood sugar imbalances, gut dysbiosis and anxiety.

How Much Fructose is Too Much?

Dr. Mercola, a renowned naturalistic physician, advises that fructose consumption should be limited to 25 mg daily for most people. For those with a high risk of or already suffering from a health condition, it would be wise to lower fructose intake to 10–15 mg daily.

How Much Fructose Are You Getting From Your Diet?

Food	Serving Size	Fructose (Grams)
Limes	1 medium	0
Lemons	1 medium	0.6
Cranberries	1 cup	0.7
Passion Fruit	1 medium	0.9
Prune	1 medium	1.2
Guava	2 medium	2.2
Date	1 medium	2.6
Cantaloupe	1/8 of medium melon	2.8
Raspberries	1 cup	3.0
Clementine	1 medium	3.4
Kiwi	1 medium	3.4
Blackberry	1 cup	3.5
Star Fruit	1 medium	3.6
Cherries (Sweet)	10	3.8
Strawberries	1 cup	3.8
Cherries (spur)	1 cup	4.0
Pineapple	1 slice	4.0

Food	Serving Size	Fructose (Grams)
Honey	1 teaspoon	4.0
Grapefruit	½ medium	4.3
Boysenberries	1 cup	4.6
Tangerine	1 medium	4.8
Nectarine	1 medium	5.4
Peach	1 medium	5.9
Orange	1 medium	6.1
Papaya	½ medium	6.3
Honeydew	1/8 of medium melon	6.7
Banana	1 medium	7.1
Blueberries	1 cup	7.4
Date (Medjool)	1 medium	7.7
Apple	1 medium	9.5
Persimmon	1 medium	10.6
Watermelon	1/16 of medium melon	11.3
Pear	1 medium	11.8
Raisins	¼ cup	12.3
Grapes	1 cup	12.4
Mango	½ medium	16.2
Apricots, dried	1 cup	16.4
Figs, dried	1 cup	23

Adapted from Mercola.com

Natural sweeteners, such as agave, honey, etc., also contain fructose, thus their consumption needs to be limited. Dr. Mercola recommends Stevia or glucose, sold as dextrose to be used instead.

So, while table sugar should not be consumed by anyone who wants to be healthy, those who suspect that they may be struggling with a bacterial or Candida overgrowth also need to limit the amount of fructose (from fruit and honey), nuts, and baked products for six to twelve weeks to starve the pathogen.

Low-Residue Fiber Diet

The low-residue fiber diet focuses on foods that are easy to digest and slow down bowel transit time. This diet is used for diverticulitis, Crohn's disease, ulcerative colitis, and bowel inflammation.

Low residue foods include meats that are well cooked and soft. Most vegetables are eaten well cooked and only a few are raw.

Juices are allowed, but only without pulp. Any vegetables with seeds should be avoided such as berries or tomatoes. Popcorn should be avoided as well.

Table 18: Low-Residue Diet: Allowed Foods

Raw Veggies	Cooked/Juiced Veggies	Fruits	Protein	Fats
Lettuce Cucumbers Onions Zucchini	Yellow squash Spinach Pumpkin Eggplant Potatoes Green beans Wax beans Asparagus Beets Carrots	Applesauce Fruit juices (no pulp) Ripe bananas, Cantaloupe Melon Papaya Peach Plums	Cooked meat Eggs Meats should be tender and soft, not chewy	Butter Oils Smooth sauces

The basic low residue fiber diet also allows bread and dairy products which are not recommended for people with Hashimoto's. Deli meats, crunchy nut butters, nuts, beans, tofu and peas are not allowed. Spicy food, chunky relishes, and chocolate are not on the diet either. Total fiber intake should be limited to 10–15 grams /day.

Trigger Removing Diets

Diets that aim to remove triggers are often helpful for reversing autoimmune conditions, but only as long as they are followed.

Dairy-free, soy-free, gluten-free, egg-free, iodine-free, Nightshade-free, and other avoidance diets have been reported to be helpful for healing Hashimoto's. Some may get better after just going gluten free, others will benefit from eliminating dairy, and others will need to eliminated a multitude of various foods.

The best practice is to follow an elimination diet to identify triggering foods instead of blindly embarking on one of these diets.

Additionally, for most, these diets may just be a remission and not a cure, unless they are combined with nourishing foods and probiotics that fix the intestinal permeability.

WHAT TO PUT IN

When we think about diets, we generally think about what we need to remove. However, the other key of a healing diet is what we add.. One can get caught up in removing various suspected foods, and still have deficiencies in beneficial bacteria and nutrients, which will prevent the thyroid and the intestines (which house the immune system) from healing.

Dietary programs focused only on what to take out are not as successful as the programs that consider what to put back in to restore optimal function.

A diet for healing Hashimoto's needs to include bone and meat broths, gelatin, protein, saturated fats, and fermented foods to help rebuild the intestinal lining. Meat, liver, and vegetable juices to help replenish depletions.

Fermented foods, such as lacto-fermented cabbage, coconut kefir (fermented coconut water), and vegetables should be at the center of this diet.

The diet should be balanced with enough vegetables to provide a healing alkaline environment.

If you were to pick just one intervention to try from this entire book, I would recommend starting to incorporate traditionally prepared fermented vegetables into your diet. Fermented vegetables are the best way to get to the root cause: unbalanced intestinal flora.

Before we had refrigerators, traditional food preparations relied on fermenting vegetables to keep them edible. Most traditional cultures ate fermented vegetables for the majority of the year. These vegetables were full of beneficial Lactobacilli bacteria that have co-evolved in a symbiotic fashion to keep us healthy. Dr. Mercola suggest that fermented cabbage may contain as much as 1 trillion colony forming units (CFUs) of beneficial microbes per serving, compared with the 10 billion CFUs per usual capsule of high-dose expensive probiotics.

Fermented vegetables are prepared by chopping the vegetables, sprinkling them with sea salt and sometimes adding water or culture starters. The vegetables are then placed in jars or other containers that can be sealed to keep air out for one to two weeks. The beneficial bacteria normally present on vegetables ferment the vegetables and create a characteristic sour taste. After the fermentation process is done, the beneficial bacteria will start dying off. Refrigeration slows down the fermentation process and thus fermented foods need to be stored in the refrigerator to preserve beneficial bacteria.

Fermented vegetables are not the same as the grocery store sauerkraut that contains vinegar and has been pasteurized to be devoid of any beneficial microflora. "Wild Fermentation" by Sandor Katz and "The Body Ecology Diet" by Donna Gates are excellent books with recipes for fermented vegetables.

Additionally, you may be able to buy raw, live fermented vegetables from farmers, health food stores, and co-ops. I order my fermented cabbage that is full of beneficial microflora from Thirty Acre Farms.

Fermented coconut meat and coconut water is also a delicious option.

I highly recommend the book Digestive Wellness by Dr. Liz Lipski for more guidance on healing diets.

Recommendations

The most comprehensive dietary approach would be as follows
1) Elemental diet for one to two weeks, followed by
2) Low-residue, low FODMAP, gut healing diet (GAPS Healing/Intro) for one to four weeks
3) Followed by an introduction diet, adding one well-cooked SCD/GAPS legal food every four days and observing for symptoms
4) Modified Full Paleo/SCD/GAPS: one to two years
5) Introduction of low-allergenic grains

The Elemental Phase would be a primarily liquid diet, with the addition of vitamin, mineral, and probiotic supplementation. This type of diet can cause weight loss, thus may not be appropriate for those who are underweight.

The second phase would introduce soups with pureed low residue vegetables, well cooked meats, juices (from mostly vegetables), gelatin, fermented coconut water, and probiotics.

The third phase would start introducing more solid foods, and may utilize digestive enzymes for meats.

General recommendations for Gut Healing Diet

Start with well-cooked foods that are easiest to digest: soups, boiled, cooked, pureed vegetables, meats. Once those are tolerated, you can add some raw pureed vegetables (I like to use the Vitamix). You can then add foods with easy to digest textures such as avocados. Continue on this way, moving forward with peeled raw fruit/vegetables and eventually advancing to eating raw vegetables with the peel.

All foods should be well cooked and ideally rotated every few days. Wait until diarrhea and flatulence stop before moving to the next level. One suggestion is to move up each level weekly, with the understanding that sometimes progression may take more or less time depending on the need of the person.

While eating raw foods is very beneficial for most people, those with leaky gut may need to avoid eating whole raw foods until the gut is well healed. Cooking vegetables makes them easier to digest, as does pureeing.

Additionally, while fiber is touted as a heath food, fiber is very hard to digest. Humans do not produce cellulase, the enzyme that is used to break down fiber, and depend on good bacteria to break down the fiber in our foods. This can be problematic in those with dysbiosis and/or SIBO, as the fiber can be fermented by the pathogenic or overgrown bacteria causing side effects and immune imbalances.

Transitioning Off the Diets.

With the exception of the Body Ecology, GAPS, Paleo, and SCD diets, most of the diets discussed in this section are healing diets and not meant to be continued long-term. Once a person stays on the diet for three months to two years, they may be able to make the transition to a less restrictive diet.

I am a big believer in diets based on traditionally prepared fermented foods, such as the one promoted by the Weston A. Price Foundation and the Body Ecology Diet. The monosaccharide diets like the GAPS, Paleo, and SCD diets are also helpful as long as they are balanced with enough veggies. My great-grandmother "Babcia Kasia", who lived on a farm in Poland and traditionally prepared all of her own foods for most of her life, was vibrant and fully capable until she died peacefully in her late 90s. A good rule of thumb may be, if your great-grandmother wouldn't eat it, you probably shouldn't eat it either. For those who come from more industrialized countries, you may need to go even beyond your great-grandmother.

For recipes and other healing resources, download the Companion Guide at www.thyroidrootcause.org/guide

Chapter Summary

✓ A personalized elimination diet should be used to determine individual intolerances.
✓ Modified monosaccharide diets are helpful for healing the gut.
✓ Elemental diet is helpful for intestinal bacterial overgrowth.

✓ Inclusion of animal protein, bone broths, fats, and fermented foods is necessary for healing.
✓ Fermented vegetables are very important, I repeat, fermented vegetables are very important!

"In order to change we must be sick and tired of being sick and tired." ~Author Unknown

19: SUPPLEMENTS

In addition to diet, supplements may be helpful with your healing journey, especially if your digestion is severely impaired, preventing you from extracting sufficient nutrients from food. You may be able to discontinue supplements once your digestion is fixed and you have adopted a well-balanced diet.

"Start Low and Go Slow"

Supplements should be started at a low dose, one at a time. Vitamins and herbs are certainly not without risks, even if they are "naturally derived." (Remember, arsenic is also a natural substance!)

You want to make sure that you start a low dose of one supplement one at a time, rather than starting the full dose of six different supplements at once. For example, you may add selenium at 200 mcg and see how you tolerate it for a few days before you decide to increase it to 400 mcg. Once you have found that you tolerate the 400 mcg dose for a few days, you can add another supplement.

Doing so will increase the likelihood of catching adverse events before they get too far and will help you pinpoint the substance that is causing you an adverse event, without having to stop all of your other supplements and delay progress.

As a clinical pharmacist, one tool I like to use is called the Naranjo Causality Scale. This tool helps to determine whether a particular substance caused an adverse event. See the modified Causality Scale on the next page.

Table 19: Modified Naranjo Causality Scale
Adapted from the Naranjo Causality Scale, 1981

	Yes	No	Don't Know
Are there previous reports on this reaction?	+1	0	0
Did the event occur after the suspected substance was administered?	+2	-1	0
Did the reaction improve after the substance was stopped, or countering substance given?	+1	0	0
Did the reaction reappear when the substance was re-given?	+2	-1	0
Are there alternative causes that could have caused this reaction?	-1	+2	0
Did the reaction occur after accidental exposure?	+1	-1	0
Was the reaction more severe when the dose was increased, or less severe when dose was decreased?	+1	0	0
Did you have a similar reaction to a similar intervention before?	+1	0	0
Was this confirmed by objective evidence (lab result, blood pressure)?	+1	0	0

Key: >8=definite, 4-7=probable, 1-3=possible, 0=doubtful

Not all Supplements are Created Equally!

Vitamin and supplement companies do not have to adhere to the same strict rules as medications in their manufacturing and labeling requirements. This leads to some supplements not having the ingredients stated on their labels or having them in doses that are either too high or too low. In some cases, they may contain substances that are not even listed on the label. Additionally, many of the excipients used in drug store brands can cause hypersensitivity reactions as well as prevent the proper absorption of the supplement.

Reports of toxicity from poorly regulated supplements are popping up every so often as well, and many brands out there are simply not worth your money or health.

Formulations Matter

Various formulations exist for mineral supplements. For example, zinc is available as zinc oxide, zinc citrate, zinc gluconate, and zinc picolinate. The picolinate formulation is the most bioavailable for zinc and chromium supplements. Taking zinc with food (after a meal) and with vitamin C increases its absorption as well.

The similar is true of ferritin. It should also be taken after meals with vitamin C.

I have researched and tried a variety of brands, and the following are the brands I recommend, and use personally.

Country Life is a gluten-, dairy-, soy- corn-, yeast-, and sugar-free brand that is sold at Whole Foods. I use selenium (L-selenomethionine 200–400 mcg), Biotin 5000 mcg and vitamin D3 5000 IU by this manufacturer.

Ortho-Molecular Products: professional-only brand that is mostly hypoallergenic. This is the only brand that carries alcohol-free licorice drops that I use every morning.

Standard Process: This is whole food nutrition company that only sells to health-care professionals. Although its products are not certified gluten/dairy free as the facility uses wheat germ to derive other products, I have used Drenatrophin PMG and Thytrophin PMG without any cross-reactivity concerns. Most of the supplements made by Standard Process are from whole food sources, which in my opinion have the best bioavailability, however the company is still working towards making the products gluten, dairy and soy free.

Rock Creek Pharmaceuticals: Anatabine lozenges, available as Anatabloc®. These supplements can be bought over the counter, however, their manufacturing process and clinical research is pharmaceutical grade. I recommend the non-flavored lozenges for those who may be sensitive to the original minty formulation. The company is currently working on additional hypoallergenic products.

Pure Encapsulations: The majority of products I use are from this company, as all of the supplements are pure, hypoallergenic, and contain no gluten, dairy or other excipients that may cause sensitivity or impair absorption. This company has extremely tight quality control procedures and each product undergoes an extensive product testing program that involves verification of label claims, potency, and purity by third-party laboratories.

Pure Encapsulations sells their products only to health-care professionals, thus patients usually have to purchase the products through their health-care providers. However, the company has allowed me to set up an E-store as a convenience for my readers, and the products I recommend and use can be viewed and purchased on thyroidrootcause.org.

I use Betaine with Pepsin, N-Acetyl-Cysteine, L-Glutamine, B_{12},

Daily Stress Formula (adrenal adaptogens), zinc picolinate and curcumin with peperine exclusively from this company. Pure Encapsulations also makes amino acids, evening primrose oil, digestive enzymes, cod liver oil, and many other high-quality products. When I go out to dinner I use their Gluten & Dairy Digest product just in the case of accidental exposures. (I have been sorry too many times after waiters were surprised that gluten was found in flour and bread: "Here's your gluten-free meal with a big piece of bread on top!") This product minimizes, but does not eliminate, the reaction I have to gluten and dairy.

Probiotics

As a pharmacologist, I always advise people to "start low and go slow" when staring supplements. This is especially true with probiotics as they can cause significant die-off symptoms that can cause further inflammation and autoimmune damage from endotoxins that are released from the dying pathogenic flora as it is displaced by the beneficial bacteria in probiotics. As people with Hashimoto's usually have low levels of alkaline phosphatase to begin with, we are not able to keep up with the daily endotoxin release from the normal life cycle of pathogenic bacteria, let alone the massive amounts that will be released when the bacteria start dying off at a fast rate.

That said, most probiotics in health food stores have maintenance doses of beneficial bacteria, doses that are too low to heal and make an impact on intestinal flora. A super-expensive high-potency probiotic may have 10 billion CFUs per capsule, while the minimal therapeutic dose for changing the gut flora is 60 billion CFUs.

For adults, I would advise starting with a 10 billion CFU dose and increasing every few days until die-off is seen.

I have tried a variety of different probiotics, and some were just a waste of money. To significantly change gut flora, I recommend only two probiotic companies.

Pure Encapsulations makes a high-quality line of multistrain probiotics with 10 billion CFUs (Probiotic-5) and a 50-billion CFU dose (Probiotic 50B). These would be a good start, but still may not be enough; depending on the degree of gut dysbiosis, the 60 billion may not even scratch the surface.

VSL #3 is a therapeutic dose, multiple strain pharmaceutical grade probiotic from Sigma-Tau Pharmaceuticals, which has been studied to improve bacterial flora and disease outcomes in ulcerative colitis and IBS. VSL #3 contains 450 billion CFUs per dose. One would need to take forty-five capsules of the brand sold in health-food stores to equal one dose of VSL #3! (At $50 for sixty capsules you would be spending $150 every four days!)

Sometimes we may even need to supplement in the trillions of CFUs. This makes sense, as the gut is home to 100 trillion bacteria, yeasts, and other microbes. For a properly functioning immune system we need a balance of approximately 85% beneficial to 15% pathogenic bacteria.

The human intestines have been found to have between 7% and 50% of Gram-negative bacteria. It is not clear how many CFUs of beneficial bacteria it takes to displace 1 CFU of pathogenic bacteria, thus while providing 1 trillion CFUs of beneficial bacteria seems like a lot, however, it may pale in comparison with the 16 trillion–50 trillion pathogenic bacteria that may be present in gut dysbiosis.

Probiotic supplements do not seem to take up residence in our intestines permanently and are described as transitional, meaning that they don't grow in the intestines. VSL#3 strains, for example, live up to three weeks in the intestines until reinforcements, in the form of additional probiotics, need to be sent in.

Caution: Many probiotics may use gluten, dairy, and soy in their manufacturing process.

Beneficial bacterial species found on raw lacto-fermented vegetables reportedly contain trillions of CFUs per dose and although not technically supplements, really are the superstars for overcoming dysbiosis and above all should be included in the healing plan.

How to get the most healing from your supplements

As a pharmacist and patient myself, I know that adherence to a medication/supplement regimen is very difficult. Adherence studies find that even when we know how to treat a condition perfectly well, in many cases when a product is recommended by a health-care professional, it does not help the patient for a variety of reasons, most of them having to do with the lack of information the patient received!

1) The patient never goes out to get the product.
2) The patient gets the wrong product, wrong dose or wrong type of medication/supplement.
3) The patient gets the correct product, but uses it incorrectly.
4) The patient gets the product and knows how to use it, but forgets to take it and uses the product only sporadically.

There is an old joke where a man goes to the doctor and says that the suppositories the doctor prescribed are not working for his constipation. Puzzled, the doctor asks "How have you been using them?" The patient replies "I swallow them, of course, what else would you do with them?"

You can spend hundreds of dollars on really great products, but if you don't use them correctly (or at all), you might as well be throwing your money away!

Some medications and supplements will not be absorbed with other supplements, or when there is food present. Others absorb better with food or other supplements. Others may need to be used at various times throughout the day due to their propensity to cause tiredness or alertness.

Thyroid hormones in particular have a lot of restrictions. They need be taken on an empty stomach, thirty minutes prior to meals, and at least four hours apart from iron, calcium, and magnesium (which can lower the absorption of the hormone).

In the transition period, you may be taking multiple supplements. It may be difficult to keep them all straight. I know it was for me. I highly recommend purchasing a pill planner. The stackable pill planners are my favorite, as they can be thrown in my purse or pockct when I need to take supplements to work or on the road. Attaching the supplements to a habit you already have (like brushing teeth, making tea) may be helpful as well. Pill reminders can be programmed to be sent to your smartphone with free apps courtesy of the pharmaceutical companies. www.mymedschedule.com

SAMPLE SUPPLEMENT SCHEDULE

<u>Morning Supplements (Best on an empty stomach)</u>

Bathroom: next to your toothbrush, take right before you brush your teeth

- ☐ Thyroid hormone (ideally wait 30 minutes until eating)
- ☐ Selenium 200-400 mcg.
- ☐ Vitamin E 400IU
- ☐ Licorice drops
- ☐ Thytrophin PMG
- ☐ Adrenal Adaptogens

Fridge, next to your breakfast foods

- ☐ Probiotics

Breakfast (put next to your tea-maker)

- ☐ Betaine with Pepsin (after protein meal)
- ☐ Glutamine powder: 5 grams in tea (it is flavorless)

Lunchtime Supplements (best with meals)

Put supplements in your lunch bag.

- ☐ Zinc Picolinate 25–50 mg
- ☐ B-Complex
- ☐ N-AcetylCysteine (NAC) 1.8 grams
- ☐ Betaine with Pepsin
- ☐ Ferritin (if your lunch is four hours or more after your morning meds)
- ☐ Fish oil
- ☐ Biotin 5000 mcg
- ☐ Vitamin D3 5000IU

Note: Take _after_ you eat. NAC will cause a stomachache without food.

Dinnertime (Best with meals)

- ☐ Betaine with Pepsin
- ☐ Ferritin (if your lunch is four hours or less after your morning meds)
- ☐ If you forgot to take your lunch supplements, you can take them at dinner, however, the B vitamins may be stimulating.

Bedtime (may be sedating)

- ☐ Magnesium

Supplement Guide

NOTE: These statements have not been evaluated by the Food and Drug Administration. The products discussed are not intended to diagnose, treat, cure, or prevent any disease

Name	Rationale	Side Effects	Notes
Adrenal adaptogens (Daily Stress Formula)	Help support adrenal function		Multiple formulations exist, cross check ingredients for sensitivities
Anatabine	Alkaloid found in tobacco, helps to detoxify LPS, reduces inflammation	May impact liver function tests. Should monitor Caution with nightshade sensitivity	Take three times-four times per day.
B_{12}	Proper development of villi, protein digestion, many others	Bright yellow urine.	Sublingual B_{12} may be better absorbed, especially is GI issues
Betaine with Pepsin	Helps digest proteins	Burning in throat, not to be used with ulcers!	Take with meals containing protein
Chromium	Required nutrient for thyroid function	May cause drowsiness	

Supplement Guide, continued

Name	Rationale	Side Effects	Notes
Curcumin	Reduces inflammation		Look for absorbable formulations
Vitamin D 5000IU	Reduce inflammation autoimmune symptoms		Ideally you should get it from the sun, but supplements can be a secondary. Can measure levels
Vitamin E 400IU	Antioxidant, works synergistically with Selenium, improves skin	Can have blood thinning effects	
Ferritin	Iron deficiency, low Ferritin levels, hair loss	May cause constipation	Wait at least 4 hours between thyroid medications. Should be taken after meals, Vitamin C, acid production helps promote absorption. *Caution with overdose

Supplement Guide, continued

Name	Rationale	Side Effects	Notes
Glutamine	Helps repair intestinal lining	Agitation	
N-Acetyl Cysteine	Helps restore gut lining, antioxidant, liver function, helps eliminate pathogenic bacteria	Stomach pain if taken on empty stomach	Take with food!
Licorice	Antiviral properties and helps stretch cortisol levels in cases of adrenal fatigue	May increase blood pressure. Avoid with high blood pressure	
Magnesium	Helps restore DHEA levels	Diarrhea, sleepiness	Becomes depleted by fluoride. Most people show deficiency.
Omega 3 or Cod Liver Oil	Reduce inflammation, improve skin condition	Can have blood thinning effects	Look for formulations free of mercury

Supplement Guide, continued

Name	Rationale	Side Effects	Notes
Probiotics or VSL #3	Lactobacillus deficiency; LB crates enzymes that aid digestion and absorption, help improve immune function, helps to balance out the pathogenic flora	Nausea, vomiting, die-off reaction	Probiotic levels can be measured by Stool tests (CDSA, GI Effects)
Proteolytic Enzymes (Systemic)	Reduce circulating immune complexes of proteins that may become antigenic		Take between meals
Saccharomyces Boulardii	Increases SIgA- helps clear out pathogenic bacteria from the body		Combine with other probiotics. Dosages higher than stated on package may need to be utilized

Supplement Guide, continued

Name	Rationale	Side Effects	Notes
Selenium 200mcg	Antioxidant, reduce TPO antibodies, helps covert T4 to T3 Will not be absorbed properly from multivitamin or Brazil nuts	Toxicity reported at excessive doses, garlic smell sign on excessive dose	Make sure to rule out Iodine deficiency. Can make hypothyroidism worse if Selenium is given in overt iodine deficiency Take on an empty stomach along with Vitamin E
Thytrophin PMG	Reduces antibodies, helps rebuild the thyroid		Dosage of up to 9 tablets per day, recheck antibodies after starting
Zinc	Required for T4 to T3 conversion Deficiency due to impaired absorption with Hashi's, Celiac, seen as low Alkaline Phosphatase on CBC	May cause copper deficiency in doses >30mg/day.	Liquid deficiency test: swish around in mouth Picolinate version is absorbed best. Take with Vitamin C and with food.

"The scientific method consists of the following steps...ask a question, do your research, construct a hypothesis, test your hypothesis, analyze your data and draw a conclusion"

20: TESTING

Lab testing, keeping track of your symptoms, basal temperatures and journaling will help you determine what problems you are having and how to address them.

Testing can help determine if your interventions are working and can help determine a course of action.

Thyroid Panel Testing

Testing TSH, Free T3 and Free T4 will help determine if you will need to have your dosage of medication adjusted.

Testing TPO antibodies every 1-3 months may be helpful in determining progress from interventions.

Food Intolerance Testing

A variety of labs offer food intolerance testing. I have heard mixed impressions from practitioners regarding these tests. The test that has been extremely reliable in my experience is the 96 and 184 panel food intolerance test offered by Alletess Medical Laboratory. I have also had great results with the ALCAT test.

Gut Function Testing

Our stool can tell quite a bit about the state of the gut. One of the most comprehensive and advanced tests is called GI Effects

Complete. This test uses DNA analysis to test the bacteria present in the gut. The test shows a balance of beneficial bacteria, parasites, markers of inflammation, digestions, absorption and sensitivity to botanicals and pharmaceuticals.

Adrenal Testing

Adrenal testing is done by collecting saliva throughout the day, and can be very helpful in identifying the stage of adrenal fatigue. These tests can also show a deficiency in Secretory IgA.

Nutrient Testing

Testing for nutrient depletions can be done through basic blood testing, by ordering specific nutrients, like Ferritin, B_{12}, etc. Hair testing may be helpful for nutrients and potentially heavy metals. SpectraCell labs offer an advanced mineral testing option.

Genetic Testing and Nutrient Extraction

Some individuals with Hashimoto's may have a gene variation that prevents them from properly activating folic acid. This gene variation is present in up to 55% of the European populations, and seems to be more common in those with hypothyroidism.

The gene involved is the MTHFR (Methylenetetrahydrofolate Reductase) gene, and genetic testing is available to show is someone has this gene variation. The MTHFR gene codes for the MTHFR enzyme, the enzyme that converts the amino acid homocysteine to methionine, a building block for proteins.

Individuals with low activity of the MTHFR enzyme may present with elevated homocysteine levels, which have been associated with inflammation and heart disease, and potentially an impaired ability to detoxify.

Nutrient deficiencies in Folate, B_6 and B_{12} have been associated with elevated homocysteine.

However, individuals with the MTHFR gene are often deficient in folate, but actually have a difficult time processing folic acid that is present in most cheap supplements and added to processed foods. Some professionals claim that this type of folic acid may even cause a build-up in the body leading to toxicity. Studies have been done that showed folic acid supplements increased cancer risk... one more reason to ditch processed foods and your multivitamin!

Folate is present in the activated form in real foods such as asparagus, spinach and beef liver, however we may not get enough of it that way. B6 and B12 are mostly found in meats.

Betaine, also known as trimethylglycine also helps with metabolizing homocysteine. Betaine can be found in whole grains like quinoa (which some individuals may not be able to eat), beets and spinach.

Individuals with the MTHFR gene variation and high homocysteine levels may benefit from an activated version of folate, B_6 and B_{12}, such as methylfolate (also known as L-5-MTHF Folate), Pyridoxyl-5-Phosphate (P5P), and methylcobalamin, respectively.

Pure Encapsulations makes a supplement called Homocysteine Factors that contains all of the above mentioned ingredients and may be helpful with reducing homocysteine levels.

TESTS AT A GLANCE

The tests in **bold** are highly recommended. Many of these tests can be ordered by your primary care physician or specialist and will be covered by most insurance plans. Optional tests are listed in plain print and may be helpful for some, but not required for all.

THYROID FUNCTION TESTS

- ☐ **TSH**
- ☐ **TPO Antibodies**
- ☐ **Thyroglobulin Antibodies**
- ☐ **Free T4**
- ☐ **Free T3**
- ☐ Reverse T3

DEPLETIONS

- ☐ **Alkaline phosphatase**
- ☐ B_{12}
- ☐ **CBC with differential**
- ☐ **Ferritin**
- ☐ **Digestive enzyme challenge**
- ☐ SpectraCell mineral testing
- ☐ Mineral hair analysis
- ☐ MTHFR gene
- ☐ Homocysteine

IMMUNE FUNCTION

- ☐ **Vitamin D levels**
- ☐ Th-1/Th-2 ratio

☐ Th-1/Th-2 stimulant challenge

INFECTION

☐ **Antibodies to viruses, bacteria, parasites**
☐ **Comprehensive Stool Test (include Yersinia)**

GUT FUNCTION

☐ Hydrogen breath test for SIBO
☐ Lactulose-Mannitol test for intestinal permeability
☐ Comprehensive stool test

ADRENAL FUNCTION

☐ **Fasting blood glucose**
☐ **Adrenal saliva profile**
☐ **Adrenal antibodies**

TRIGGERS

☐ **My timeline**
☐ **Iodine intake assessment**
☐ Iodine urine test

INTOLERANCES

☐ **Elimination diet**
☐ IgA food intolerance screen
☐ IgG food sensitivity panel
☐ ALCAT

TOXINS

☐ **Liver function tests**
☐ **Assessment**
☐ Mineral hair analysis

Work with your practitioner to order the appropriate lab tests to help guide your treatment plan.

Always be sure to get a copy of your own test results so that you have an opportunity to see what's going on and do your own research.

Patient Self-Order Lab Testing Companies

In the case that you are unable to find a provider that will perform the necessary lab tests for you, some companies provide direct-to-consumer lab testing. I have successfully used the following companies:

My Labs For Life-offers access to a variety of blood tests including alkaline phosphatase, TPO Antibodies, celiac panel, PCB Exposure, reverseT3, Selenium, CBC, MTHFR gene variation, food sensitivity panel. Patients can order their own lab tests and are sent to LabCorp locations for blood draws. www.mylabsforlife.com

My Med Lab- this lab has a panel of tests including a thyroid panel, GI Effects Complete and saliva adrenal testing www.mymedlab.com

ZRT Labs allows patients to order their own labs. All blood tests done through non-invasive saliva, urine or blood spot testing. Available tests include TSH, free T3, TPO antibodies and urinary iodine www.zrtlab.com

**These companies do not require a physician's order to perform lab testing.

Appendix: My Timeline

- **START:** Age 3: April 29, 1986: Chernobyl disaster in Ukraine; (lived close to Ukraine border, received iodine)

- 1994: Began menses, mother concerned about my thyroid because I was very thin and had an enlarged thyroid gland, took to endocrinologist in Poland while on vacation. Tests showed that I was "euthyroid" (had normal thyroid levels).

- 1996–2000: high school, energetic (busy bee), only required six to eight hours of sleep, never took naps. Was on honor roll, in extracurricular activities, part-time job, rarely sick except for bronchitis freshman year. Started smoking five cigarettes a day, still very thin, took "GNC Weight Gainer" every few months to help with weight maintenance.

- 2000: Started college, University of Illinois; recurrent strep throat infections treated with antibiotics. Started oral contraceptives for severe menstrual cramps.

- April–May? 2001: Poor energy, sore throat, and swollen lymph nodes. Diagnosed with strep throat by university clinic right before finals. Went on to sleep sixteen-plus hours per day with depressed mood, inability to make decisions, decreased concentration. Later diagnosed with mononucleosis (EBV) after complaining of swollen lymph node on left side of neck with occasional sharp stabbing pains. Never fully recovered from the increased sleep requirement, needing ten-plus hours of sleep and decreased ability to concentrate. Was down to 92 pounds (received flu shot for first time that year as well).

- 2002–03: woke up with severe, explosive diarrhea with cramping after eating ramen noodles containing soy the night before. This pattern repeated for less than a year, almost daily (three times week) usually after eating. Led to needing to carry a sh*t kit at all times (Imodium, Pepto Bismol, baby wipes). Diagnosed with IBS, later asked pharmacist if it could be intolerant to Ensure or morning shakes, and she advised to avoid "soy lecithin." Diarrhea frequency reduced after avoiding soy lecithin containing products, however still occasionally occurred (once a week to once a month).

- September 2005: treated with antibiotics, antifungals for infections

- March 2006: Graduated Pharmacy school, got engaged, was moving out of state. Started to have severe anxiety. Lots of changes that made me feel stressed out. Decided to stop drinking Red Bull, with some improvement.

- August 2006: Moved to Phoenix, Ariz., living for the first time on my own, away from everyone I knew. I noticed my hair was really tangled, difficult to brush. Blamed the water.

- 2006: Feeling tired but happy, had physical to determine cause of being tired. Everything was "normal."

- 2006: received antibiotics for acne

- 2007: read "The Abs Diet" and started drinking whey protein shakes in preparation for wedding

- January 2008: contracted severe infection with cough and chest pain, not helped by over-the-counter cough meds, got prescription for Phenergan with codeine, diagnosed as viral

- Sometime in 2008 had recurrent infection, treated with metronidazole, clindamycin, and doxycycline

- March 2008: despite resolution of infection, cough persisted.- uncontrollable, with tearing eyes, petechiae on neck, sometimes to the point of vomiting. Woke up in middle of night choking, would cough when talking to people, when eating. Tried all OTC cough medications, antihistamines, etc. Went back to clinic, diagnosed allergies/post-nasal drip. Did not feel I had allergies. Suspected asthma because of mother's and aunt's asthma developed in their 20s and 30s. Tried Singulair in addition to other meds, with limited help.

- July 2008: decided to find better PCP for chronic cough. Doctor ran chest X-ray (came out negative); allergy panel, etc. TSH was slightly elevated at 4.5 (MD said thyroid was normal). MD blamed chronic cough on allergies. He recommended air purifier.

- August 2008: saw allergist based on allergy panel (tested positive for dogs). She suspected GERD and referred to GI specialist for barium swallow. Also diagnosed allergies. Ran thyroid antibodies test=2000+. TSH and FT4 were "normal," according to old reference ranges. She informed me I'm at risk for Hashimoto's, but did not explain relevance.

- September 2008: GI diagnosed reflux, (silent), because no symptoms. Took allergy (Singulair) and reflux medication (PPI) despite having no symptoms of either besides the chronic cough until Dec 2008. Cough continued with new onset of reflux symptoms (burping, burning, chest pain)

- January 2009: decided to discontinue PPI and allergy meds. Started self on Pepcid and removed beans, tomato juice, lemons, and oranges from diet. Symptoms improved 80%, however, still had occasional coughing outbursts. Used Mylanta for occasional symptom relief. Felt like gag reflex was oversensitive ...

- March 2009: Started having sharp stabbing pain in ears, also coughed whenever put Q-tip in left ear (bizarre); wondered if tonsilloliths contributed to gag reflex and coughing. Saw ear, nose, and throat specialist who wanted to remove tonsils, but had no clue about stabbing ear pain.

- June 2009: traveled to Poland and Germany. Had delicious food, and unfortunately food poisoning multiple times per day. Also had hives, lip itching, allergies, and reflux.

- July–August 2009: started noticing hair loss—diffuse, much more hair in tub, every time I run hand through hair, wash it, and touch it! (Now probably have less 60–70% of hair I had.)

- September 2009: visit with PCP for annual checkup: TSH=7.95, (normal T4), Diagnosis: Hashimoto's Thyroiditis, subclinical hypothyroidism, suspected mitral valve prolapse, murmur. Referred to cardiologist, endocrinologist.

END OF TIMELINE

References

Chapter 1 References

1. Gärtner R, Gasnier BC, Dietrich JW, Krebs B, Angstwurm MW. Selenium supplementation in patients with autoimmune thyroiditis decreases thyroid peroxidase antibodies concentrations. J Clin Endocrinol Metab. 2002 Apr;87(4):1687-91
2. Mcdermott M.T., Ridgway C.: Subclinical hypothyroidism is mild thyroid failure and should be treated. J Clin Endocrinol Met 86. (10): 4585-4590.2001
3. Sategna-Guidetti C, Volta U, Ciacci C, Usai P, Carlino A, De Franceschi L, Camera A, Pelli A, Brossa C. Prevalence of thyroid disorders in untreated adult celiac disease patients and effect of gluten withdrawal: an Italian multicenter study. Am J Gastroenterol. 2001 Mar;96(3):751-7.
4. http://www.thyroid-info.com/topdrs/california2.htm accessed on 5/1/2013

Chapter 2 References

1. Davies, TF. Pathogenesis of Hashimoto's thyroiditis (chronic autoimmune thyroiditis) Ross, DS. UpToDate
2. 2012 Clinical Practice Guidelines for Hypothyroidism in Adults: Available at http://aace.metapress.com/content/b67v7mk73g3233n2/fulltext.pdf
3. Ahad F, Ganie SA. Iodine, Iodine metabolism and Iodine deficiency disorders revisited. Indian J Endocrinol Metab. 2010 Jan-Mar; 14(1): 13–17.
4. Müssig K, Künle A, Säuberlich AL, Weinert C, Ethofer T, Saur R, Klein R, Häring HU, Klingberg S, Gallwitz B, Leyhe T. Thyroid peroxidase antibody positivity is associated with symptomatic distress in patients with Hashimoto's thyroiditis. Brain Behav Immun. 2012 May;26(4):559-63. doi: 10.1016/j.bbi.2012.01.006. Epub 2012 Jan 21.
5. Neck Check Card. Accessed at healingdeva.com/NeckCheckCard.pdf on 2/22/13
6. The Merck Manual of Medical Information - Second Home Edition, p. 948, edited by Mark H. Beers. Copyright © 2003 by Merck & Co., Inc., Whitehouse Station, NJ. Available at: http://www.merck.com/mmhe/sec13/ch163/ch163a.html Accessed March 29, 2013
7. Carta MG, Loviselli A, Hardoy MC, Massa S, Cadeddu M, Sardu C, Carpiniello B, Dell'Osso L, Mariotti S. The link between thyroid autoimmunity (antithyroid peroxidase autoantibodies) with anxiety and mood disorders in the community: a field of interest for public health in the future. BMC Psychiatry. 2004 Aug 18;4:25.
8. Takasu N et al. Test for recovery from hypothyroidism during thyroxine therapy in Hashimoto's thyroiditis. *Lancet* 1990 Nov 3 336 1084-1086

9.   Cooper R, Lerer B. The use of thyroid hormones in the treatment of depression] Harefuah. 2010 Aug;149(8):529-34, 550, 549
10. Barbesino G. Drugs affecting thyroid function Thyroid. 2010 Jul;20(7):763-70
11. Gaynes BM, et. al. The STAR*D study: Treating depression in the real world. Cleveland Clinic Journal of Medicine. 75 (1), Jan 2008, 57-66.
12. Nanan R, Wall JR. Remission of Hashimoto's Thyroiditis in a twelve-year-old girl with thyroid changes documented by ultrasonography. Thyroid 20(10), 2010
13. What is Thyroiditis? American Thyroid Association. Accessed on 5/1/2013 at http://thyroid.org/what-is-thyroiditis/
14. Akamizu T, Amino N, De Groot L. Chapter 8-Hashimoto's Thyroiditis. Accessed on 4/1/2012 at www.thyroidmanager.org
15. Ross DS. Thyroid Hormone Synthesis and physiology. UpToDate; 2013
16. Klein RZ, Sargent JD, Larsen PR, Waisbren SE, Haddow JE, Mitchell ML. Relation of severity of maternal hypothyroidism to cognitive development of offspring. J Med Screen, 2001; 8(1): 18-20
17. Sarkar, D. Recurrent pregnancy loss in patients with thyroid dysfunction. Indian J Endocrinol Metab. 2012 Dec; 16 (Suppl 2)
18. Khalid AS, Joyce C, O'Donoghue K. Prevalence of subclinical and undiagnosed overt hypothyroidism in a pregnancy loss clinic. Ir Med J. 2013 Apr; 106(4): 107-10

Chapter 3 References

1.   Tirosint website www.tirosint.com/ accessed on 2/22/13
2.   Thyrolar Website www.thyrolar.com accessed on 1/20/13
3.   Ito S, Tamura T, Nishikawa M. Effects of desiccated thyroid, prednisolone and chloroquine on goiter and antibody titer in chronic thyroiditis. Metabolism 17:317, 1968.
4.   Jonklaas J, Talbert RL. Chapter 84. Thyroid Disorders. In: Talbert RL, DiPiro JT, Matzke GR, Posey LM, Wells BG, Yee GC, eds. Pharmacotherapy: A Pathophysiologic Approach. 8th ed. New York: McGraw-Hill; 2011.
5.   Takasu N, Komiya I, Asawa T, Nagasawa Y, Yamada T. Test for recovery from hypothyroidism during thyroxine therapy in Hashimoto's thyroiditis. Lancet. 1990 Nov 3;336(8723):1084-6.
6.   Haskell, ND. Hope for Hashimoto's , Advancing Medical Care Inc. 2011
7.   http://www.21centurymed.com/?page_id=474 accessed 5/1/2013
8.   http://www.clinicaltrials.gov/ct2/results?term=NCT01739972&Search= Search
9.   Brownstein D. Overcoming Thyroid Disorders 2nd edition. Medical Alternative's Press. 2008
10. 2012 Clinical Practice Guidelines for Hypothyroidism in Adults: Available at http://aace.metapress.com/content/b67v7mk73g3233n2/fulltext.pdf

11. Mcdermott M.T., Ridgway C.: Subclinical hypothyroidism is mild thyroid failure and should be treated. J Clin Endocrinol Met 86. (10): 4585-4590.2001
12. http://www.npthyroid.com
13. Hoang TD, et. al. Desiccated thyroid extract compared with levothyroxine in the treatment of hypothyroidism: a randomized, double-blind, crossover study.J Clin Endocrinol Metab. 2013 May;98(5):1982-90

Chapter 4 References

1. Fasano A. Leaky Gut and autoimmune disease. Clin Rev Allergy Immunol. 2012 Feb;42(1):71-8.
2. Fasano A. Zonulin and Its Regulation of Intestinal Barrier Function: The Biological Door to Inflammation, Autoimmunity, and Cancer. Physiol Rev. Vol 91. Jan 2011. 151-175
3. Ahad F, Ganie SA. Iodine metabolism and Iodine deficiency disorders revisited. Indian J Endocrinol Metab. 2010 Jan-Mar; 14(1): 13–17.
4. Strieder TGA, Tijssen JGP, Wenzel BE, Endert E, Wiersinga WM. Prediction of Progression to Overt Hypothyroidism or Hyperthyroidism in female relatives of patients with autoimmune thyroid diseases using the Thyroid Events Amsterdam (THEA) Score. Arch Intern Med/Vol 168 (No 15), Aug 11/25, 2008
5. Suen RM, Gordon S. A Critical Review of IgG Immunoglobulins and Food Allergy-Implications in Systemic Health. Us BioTek Laboratories, 2003
6. Davies, TF. Pathogenesis of Hashimoto's thyroiditis (chronic autoimmune thyroiditis) Ross, DS. UpToDate
7. https://www.standardprocess.com/Products/Standard-Process/Thytrophin-PMG accessed 5/1/13

Chapter 5 References

1. Nanan R, Wall JR. Remission of Hashimoto's Thyroiditis in a twelve-year-old girl with thyroid changes documented by ultrasonography. Thyroid 20(10), 2010

Chapter 6 References

1. Cohen S. Drug Muggers. Rodale. 2011
2. Nutrient Depletions in Natural Standard: the authority on integrative medicine [database on the Internet]. Cambridge (MA): Natural Standard; 2012 [cited 5 December 2012]. Available from: http://www.naturalstandard.com. Subscription required to view.
3. Shrader SP, Diaz VA. Chapter 88. Contraception. In: Talbert RL, DiPiro JT, Matzke GR, Posey LM, Wells BG, Yee GC, eds. Pharmacotherapy: A Pathophysiologic Approach. 8th ed. New York: McGraw-Hill; 2011. http://0-

www.accesspharmacy.com.millennium.midwestern.edu/content.aspx?aID
=7993297. Accessed May 4, 2013.

4. Daher R, Yazbeck T, Bou Jaoude J, Abboud B. Consequences of dysthyroidism on the digestive tract and viscera. World J Gastroenterol 2009; 15(23): 2834-2838 Available from: URL: http://www.wjgnet.com/1007-9327/15/2834.asp

5. Wada L, King JC. Effect of low zinc intakes on basal metabolic rate, thyroid hormones and protein utilization in adult men. J Nutr 1986;116:1045–53.

6. Sategna-Guidetti C, Volta U, Ciacci C, Usai P, Carlino A, De Franceschi L, Camera A, Pelli A, Brossa C. Prevalence of thyroid disorders in untreated adult celiac disease patients and effect of gluten withdrawal: an Italian multicenter study. Am J Gastroenterol. 2001 Mar;96(3):751-7.

7. Dietary Supplement Fact Sheet: Selenium. National Institute of Health. Office of Dietary Supplements. http://ods.od.nih.gov/factsheets/Selenium-HealthProfessional/ Accessed 8/1/12

8. FAO Document Repository-Selenium. Available at http://www.fao.org/docrep/004/Y2809E/y2809e0l.htm Accessed 8/2/12

9. Longnecker MP, Taylor PR, Levander OA, Howe M, Veillon C, McAdam PA, Patterson KY, Holden JM, Stampfer MJ, Morris JS, et al. Selenium in diet, blood, and toenails in relation to human health in a seleniferous area. Am J Clin Nutr. 1991 May;53(5):1288 94.

10. Balazs C, Kaczur V. Effect of Selenium on HLA-DR Expression of Thyrocytes. Autoimmune Dis. 2012; 2012: 374635 PMCID: PMC3286896

11. Hope for Hashimoto's

12. Gärtner R, Gasnier BC, Dietrich JW, Krebs B, Angstwurm MW. Selenium supplementation in patients with autoimmune thyroiditis decreases thyroid peroxidase antibodies concentrations. J Clin Endocrinol Metab. 2002 Apr;87(4):1687-91.

13. (Fan AM, Kizer KW: Selenium-Nutritional, toxicologic, and clinical aspects. West J Med 1990 Aug; 153:160-167)

14. Negro, R. Selenium and thyroid autoimmunity. Biologics, 2008 June, 2 (2): 265-273 PMC2721352

15. Xu J, Liu XL, Yang XF, Guo HL, Zhao LN, Sun XF.Supplemental selenium alleviates the toxic effects of excessive iodine on thyroid. Biol Trace Elem Res. 2011 Jun;141(1-3):110-8. Epub 2010 Jun 2.

16. Contempre B, Dumont JE, Ngo B, Thilly CH, Diplock AT, Vanderpas J.J Clin Endocrinol Metab. 1991 Jul;73(1):213-5. Effect of selenium supplementation in hypothyroid subjects of an iodine and selenium deficient area: the possible danger of indiscriminate supplementation of iodine-deficient subjects with selenium.

17. Chang JC, Gutenmann WH, Reid CM, Lisk DJ, Selenium content of Brazil nuts from two geographic locations in Brazil. Chemosphere. 1995 Feb; 30(4). 801-802

18. Tolonen M, Taipale M, Viander B, Pihlava JM, Korhonen H, Ryhänen EL. Plant-derived biomolecules in fermented cabbage. J Agric Food Chem. 2002 Nov 6;50(23):6798-803.
19. Fort, P (04/1990). "Breast and soy-formula feedings in early infancy and the prevalence of autoimmune thyroid disease in children". Journal of the American College of Nutrition (0731-5724), 9 (2), 164.
20. Medeiros-Neto, Geraldo (03/2012). "Approach to and treatment of goiters". The Medical clinics of North America (0025-7125), 96 (2), 351.
21. Doerge DR, Chang HC. Inactivation of thyroid peroxidase by soy isoflavones, in vitro and in vivo. J Chromatogr B Analyt Technol Biomed Life Sci 2002;777: 269–79.

Chapter 7 References

2. Iodine. Inchem. http://www.inchem.org/documents/jecfa/jecmono/v024je11.htm Accessed 8/1/12
3. Iodine Content of Foods. http://foodhealth.info/iodine/ Accessed 8/1/12
4. Abraham, G.E, MD, Facts about Iodine and Autoimmune Thyroiditis The Original Internist, Vol. 15, No. 2, pg. 75-76, June 2008
5. Dietary Supplement Fact Sheet: Iodine . National Institute of Health. Office of Dietary Supplements http://ods.od.nih.gov/factsheets/Iodine-HealthProfessional/ Accessed 8/1/12
6. Zimmerman MB. Iodine deficiency. Endocr Rev. 2009 Jun;30(4):376-408. Epub 2009 May 21.
7. Reinhardt W, Luster M, Rudorff KH, Heckmann C, Petrasch S, Lederbogen S, et al. Effect of small doses of iodine on thyroid function in patients with Hashimoto's thyroiditis residing in an area of mild iodine deficiency. Eur J Endocrinol. 1998;139:23–8. doi: 10.1530/eje.0.1390023. [PubMed] [Cross Ref]
8. Heydarian P, Ordookhani A, Azizi F. Goiter rate, serum thyrotropin, thyroid autoantibodies and urinary iodine concentration in Tehranian adults before and after national salt iodization. J Endocrinol Invest. 2007;30:404–10. [PubMed]
9. Doufas AG, Mastorakos G, Chatziioannou S, Tseleni-Balafouta S, Piperingos G, Boukis MA, et al. The predominant form of non-toxic goiter in Greece is now autoimmune thyroiditis. Eur J Endocrinol. 1999;140:505–11. doi: 10.1530/eje.0.1400505. [PubMed] [Cross Ref]
10. Lind P, Kumnig G, Heinisch M, Igerc I, Mikosch P, Gallowitsch HJ, et al. Iodine supplementation in Austria: methods and results. Thyroid. 2002;12:903–7. doi: 10.1089/105072502761016539. [PubMed] [Cross Ref
11. Stazi AV, Trinti B. [Selenium deficiency in celiac disease: risk of autoimmune thyroid diseases].Minerva Med. 2008 Dec;99(6):643-53.
12. Murray CW, Egan SK, Kim H, Beru N, Bolger PM. US Food and Drug Administration's Total Diet Study: dietary intake of perchlorate and

iodine.J Expo Sci Environ Epidemiol. 2008 Nov;18(6):571-80. Epub 2008 Jan 2.

13. Zaletel, K, Gaberscek S, Pirnat E, Krhin B, Hojker S. Ten-year follow-up of thyroid epidemiology in Slovenia after increase in salt iodization. Croat Med J. 2011 October; 52(5): 615–621.

14. Yoon, S, Choi S, Kim D, Kim J, Kim K, Ahm C, Cha B, Lim S, Kim K, Lee H, Huh K. The Effect of Iodine Restriction on Thyroid Function in Patients with Hypothyroidism Due to Hashimoto's Thyroiditis. Yonsei Medical Journal, Vol.44, No. 2. Pp.227-235; 2003

15. Xue H, Wang W, Li Y, Shan Z, Li Y, Teng X, Gao Y, Fan C, Teng W.Selenium upregulates CD4(+)CD25(+) regulatory T cells in iodine-induced autoimmune thyroiditis model of NOD.H-2(h4) mice. Endocr J. 2010;57(7):595-601. Epub 2010 Apr 27

16. N R Rose, L Rasooly, A M Saboori, and C L Burek. Linking iodine with autoimmune thyroiditis. Environ Health Perspect. 1999 October; 107(Suppl 5): 749–752. PMCID: PMC1566262 (about T cell proliferation)

17. Haskell, ND. Hope for Hashimoto's , Advancing Medical Care Inc. 2011

18. Mazziotti G, Premawardhana LDKE, Parkes AB, Adams H, Smuth PPA, Smith DF, Kaluarachi WN, Wijeyaratne CN, Jayasinghe A, de Silva DGH, Lazarus JH. Evolution of thyroid autoimmunity during iodine prophylazis-the Sri Lankan experiences. European Journal of Endocrinology (2003) 149; 103-110

19. Taskforce for Iodinization

20. Laurberg P, Cerqueira C, Ovesen L, Rasmussen LB, Perrild H, Andersen S, Pedersen IB, Carlé A.Iodine intake as a determinant of thyroid disorders in populations. Best Pract Res Clin Endocrinol Metab. 2010 Feb;24(1):13-27.

21. Zava TT, Zava DT Assessment of Japanese iodine intake based on seaweed consumption in Japan: A literature-based analysis. *Thyroid Research* 2011, 4:14

22. Large Differences in Incidences of Overt Hyper- and Hypothyroidism Associated with a Small Difference in Iodine Intake: A Prospective Comparative Register-Based Population Survey J. Clin. Endocrinol. Metab. 2002 87: 4462-4469

23. Chistiakov DA. Immunogenetics of Hashimoto's thyroiditis. J Autoimmune Dis. 2005; 2: 1.

24. http://www.centrum.com/centrum-adults-under-50#tablets assessed on 10/3/12

25. www.penncancer.org/pdf/education/LowIodineDiet.pdf assessed on 10/3/12

26. Low Iodine Diet Cookbook. 2010 ThyCa: Thyroid Cancer Survivors' Association, Inc Available at: http://thyca.org/Cookbook.pdf assessed on 10/4/12

27. http://thyroid.about.com/gi/o.htm?zi=1/XJ&zTi=1&sdn=thyroid&cdn =health&tm=13&f=12&su=p284.13.342.ip_&tt=2&bt=1&bts=1&zu=ht tp%3A//www.thyroid-info.com/articles/brownstein-hormones.htm

28. Pedersen IB, Knudsen N, Jorgensen T, Perrild H, Oversen L, Laurberg P. Large Differences in Incidences of Overt Hyper- and Hypothyroidism Associated with a Small Difference in Iodine Intake: A Prospective Comparative Register- Based Population Survey. The Journal of Clinical Endocrinology & Metabolism October 1, 2002 vol. 87 no. 10 4462-4469

29. Okamura K, Ueda K, Sone H, Ikenoue H, Hasuo Y, Sato K, Yoshinary M, Fujishima M. A sensitive thyroid hormone assay for screening a thyroid functional disorder in elderly Japanese. J Am Geriatr Soc. 1989;37:317–322

Chapter 8 References

1. Maes M, Mihaylova I, Leunis JC.In chronic fatigue syndrome, the decreased levels of omega-3 poly-unsaturated fatty acids are related to lowered serum zinc and defects in T cell activation. Neuro Endocrinol Lett. 2005 Dec;26(6):745-51.

2. Simopoulos AP. The importance of the ratio of omega-6/omega-3 essential fatty acids. Biomed Pharmacother. 2002 Oct;56(8):365-79.

Chapter 9 References

1. Davies, T. Ross D, Mulder JE. Pathogenesis of Hashimoto's thyroiditis (chronic autoimmune thyroiditis). UptoDate

2. Morohoshi K, Takahashi Y, Mori K. Viral infection and innate pattern recognition receptors in induction of Hashimoto's thyroiditis. Discov Med. 2011 Dec;12(67):505-11.

3. Penna G et.al. Vitamin D Receptor Agonists in the Treatment of Autoimmune Diseases: Selective Targeting of Myeloid but Not Plasmacytoid Dendritic Cells. J Bone Miner Res 2007;22:V69–V73

4. Diagnosis of Parasitic Diseases. Centers for Disaese Control . Accessed at: www.cdc.gov/parasites/references_resources/diagnosis.html on 2/8/13

5. Parasite detected in a patient suffering with Hashimoto's. Accessed on 2/8/13 at: http://www.drhagmeyer.com/hypothyroidism/thyroid-disease-parasites-are-often-found-can-this-be-part-of-your-problem/

6. Keynan Y, et.al. The Role of Regulatory T Cells in Chronic and Acute Viral Infections. Clin Infect Dis. (2008) 46 (7):1046-1052.

7. Maes M, Twisk FN, Kubera M, Ringel K, Leunis JC, Geffard M. Increased IgA responses to the LPS of commensal bacteria is associated with inflammation and activation of cell-mediated immunity in chronic fatigue syndrome.J Affect Disord. 2012 Feb;136(3):909-17 2.

8. Hierholzer, JC, Kabara, JJ. In vitro effects of monolaurin compounds on enveloped RNA and DNA viruses. Journal of Food Safety, 4:1, 1982.

9. http://www.umm.edu/altmed/articles/intestinal-parasites-000097.htm

10. Maes M, Leunis JC. Normalization of leaky gut in chronic fatigue syndrome (CFS) is accompanied by a clinical improvement: effects of age, duration of illness and the translocation of LPS from gram-

negative bacteria. Neuro Endocrinol Lett. 2008 Dec;29(6):902-10

11. Okeniyi JA, Ogunlesi TA, Oyelami OA, Adeyemi LA. Effectiveness of dried Carica papaya seeds against human intestinal parasitosis: a pilot study. J Med Food. 2007;10(1):194-6.

12. "Incidences of antibodies to Yersinia enterocolitica: high incidence of serotype O5 in autoimmune thyroid diseases in Japan"; Asari S, Amino N, Horikawa M, Miyai K.; Central Laboratory for Clinical Investigation, Osaka University Medical School, Japan.

13. "Association of Parvovirus B19 Infection and Hashimoto's Thyroiditis in Children"; Hartwig W. Lehmann, Nicola Lutterbüse, Annelie Plentz, Ilker Akkurt, Norbert Albers, Berthold P. Hauffa, Olaf Hiort, Eckhard Schoenau, Susanne Modrow. Viral Immunology. September 2008, 21(3): 379-384. doi:10.1089/vim.2008.0001.

14. Caselli E, Zatelli MC, Rizzo R, Benedetti S, Martorelli D, et al. (2012) Virologic and Immunologic Evidence Supporting an Association between HHV-6 and Hashimoto's Thyroiditis. PLoS Pathog 8(10):

15. Lin, JC. Antiviral Therapy for Epstein-Barr Virus-Associated Diseases. Tzu Chi Med J 2005; 17:1-10

16. Sisto M. et.al. Proposing a relationship between Mycobacterium avium subspecies paratuberculosis infection and Hashimoto's thyroiditis. Scandinavian Journal of Infectious Diseases, 2010; 42: 787–790

17. Guarneri F, et.al. Bioinformatics Support the Possible Triggering of Autoimmune Thyroid Diseases by Yersinia enterocolitica Outer Membrane Proteins Homologous to the Human Thyrotropin Receptor. THYROID . Volume 21, Number 11, 2011

18. Blanco, JL, Garcia ME. Immune response to fungal infections. Veterinary Immunology and Immunopathology 125 (2008) 47–70

19. Amin OM, Amin KO. Herbal Remedies for Parasitic Infections. Explore! Volume 8, number 6, 1998. Addendum accessed at www.parasitetesting.com/ on 2/8/13

20. Albert PJ, Proal AD, Marshall TG. Vitamin D: the alternative hypothesis. Autoimmunity Reviews, 2009

21. Hesham, MS. Intestinal parasitic infections and micronutrient deficiency: a review. Medical journal of Malaysia (0300-5283), 59 (2), 284.

22. thyroid.about.com/library/weekly/aa042301.htm accessed10/11/12

23. http://www.siboinfo.com accessed 10/13/12

24. Brownstein D. Overcoming Thyroid Disorders 2nd edition. Medical Alternative's Press. 2008

25. Greenstein RJ, Su L, Brown ST.. The Thioamides Methimazole and Thiourea Inhibit Growth of M. avium Subspecies paratuberculosis in Culture. PLoS One. 2010 Jun 14;5(6):e11099.

26. Sands, J, et al. Extreme sensitivity of enveloped viruses, including Herpes Simplex, to long chain unsaturated monoglycerides and alcohols, Antimicrobial Agents and Chemotherapy. 15; 1:67-73, 1979.

27. Pender MP. Cd8+ T-cell deficiency, Epstein-Barr virus infection, Vitamin D deficiency, and steps to autoimmunity: A unifying hypothesis. Autoimmune diseases Volume 2012, Article ID 189096

28. Penna G, Amuchastegui S, Laverny G, Adorini L. Vitamin D Receptor Agonists in the Treatment Diseases; Selective Targeting of the myeloid but not plasmacytoid dendric cells. J Bone Miner Res 2007; 22: V69-V73

Chapter 10 References

1. Nanba T, Watanabe M, Inoue N, Iwatani Y. Increases of the Th1/Th2 Cell Ratio in Severe Hashimoto's Disease and in the Proportion of TH17 Cells in Intractable Graves' Disease. Thyroid. 2009 May;19(5):495-501.

2. Phenekos C, Vryonidou A, Gritzapis AD, Baxevanis CN, Goula M, Papamichail M.Th1 and Th2 serum cytokine profiles characterize patients with Hashimoto's thyroiditis (Th1) and Graves' disease (Th2). Neuroimmunomodulation. 2004;11(4):209-13.

3. Wilder RL. Adrenal and gonadal steroid hormone deficiency in the pathogenesis of rheumatoid arthritis. J Rheumatol Suppl. 1996 Mar;44:10-2

4. HiroseY, Murosaki S, YamamotoY, YoshikaiY, Tsuru T. Daily Intake of Heat-Killed Lactobacillus plantarum L-137 Augments Acquired Immunity in Healthy Adults. J. Nutr. 136: 3069–3073, 2006.

5. Issazadeh-Navikas S, Teimer R, Bockermann R. Influence of Dietary Components on Regulatory T Cells. MOL MED 18:95-110, 2012

6. Wong CP, Nguyen LP, Noh SK, Braya TM, Bruno RS, Ho E. Induction of regulatory T cells by green tea polyphenol EGCG. Immunol Lett (2011), doi:10.1016/j.imlet.2011.04.009

7. Lactobacillus Plantarum: The Key Benefits of this "Superstar" Probiotic & How to Get It In Your Diet. Body Ecology. Accessed at: http://bodyecology.com/articles/lactobacillus_plantarum_benefits.php accessed on 11/1/12

8. Fang SP, Tanaka T, Tago F, Okamoto T, Kojima S. Immunomodulatory effects of gyokuheifusan on INF-gamma/IL-4 (Th1/Th2) balance in ovalbumin (OVA)-induced asthma model mice. Biol Pharm Bull. 2005 May;28(5):829-33.

9. Giron-Gonzalez JA, Moral FJ, Elvira J, Garcia-Gil D, Guerrero F, Gavilan, Escobar L. Consistent production of a higher TH1:TH2 cytokine ratio by stimulated T cells in men compared with women. European Journal of Endocrinology (2000) 143 31-36

10. Gonzalez S, Alcaraz MV, Cuevas J, Perez M, Jaen P, Alvarez-Mon M, Villarrubia VG. An extract of the fern Polypodium leucotomos (Difur) modulates Th1/Th2 cytokines balance in vitro and appears to exhibit anti-angiogenic activities in vivo: pathogenic relationships and therapeutic implications. Anticancer Res. 2000 May-Jun;20(3A):1567-75.

11. Fraternale A, Paoletti MF, Casabianca A, Oiry J, Clayette P, Vogel JU, Cinatl J Jr, Palamara AT, Sgarbanti R, Garaci E, Millo E, Benatti U, Magnani M.

Antiviral and immunomodulatory properties of new pro-glutathione (GSH) molecules. Curr Med Chem. 2006;13(15):1749-55.

12. Fraternale A, Paoletti MF, Casabianca A, Oiry J, Clayette P, Vogel JU, Cinatl J Jr, Palamara AT, Sgarbanti R, Garaci E, Millo E, Benatti U, Magnani M. Antiviral and immunomodulatory properties of new pro-glutathione (GSH) molecules.

13. Is Your Immune System Out of Whack? Find Out How to Avoid Dietary Triggers That May Be Causing Serious Health Problems! Body Ecology. Accessed at: http://bodyecology.com/articles/immune-system-dietary-triggers-health-problems.php 11/1/12

14. Kidd, P. TH1/Th2 Balance: The Hypothesis, its Limitations, and Implications for Health and Disease. Alternative Medicine Review. Volume 8, Number 3. 223-246. 2003

15. Th1 vs Th2 And Autoimmunity. Alkylosing Spondylitis Research Diet. Accessed on 11/1/12 at: http://sites.google.com/site/cureankylosingspondylitis/research/th1-vs-th2-and-autoimmunity

16. Maureen W. Groer and Mitzi W. Davis. Cytokines, Infections, Stress, and Dysphoric Moods in Breastfeeders and Formula feeders. Journal of Obstetric, Gynecologic, and Neonatal Nursing. 35, 599-607; 2006.

17. Abdullah M, Chai PS, Loh CY, Chong MY, Quay HW, Vidyadaran S, Seman Z, Kandiah M, Seow HF. Carica papaya increases regulatory T cells and reduces IFN-γ+ CD4+ T cells in healthy human subjects. Mol Nutr Food Res. 2011 May;55(5):803-6. doi: 10.1002/mnfr.201100087. Epub 2011 Mar 24.

18. Horrigan LA, Kelly JP, Connor TJ. Immunomodulatory effects of caffeine: friend or foe? Pharmacol Ther. 2006 Sep;111(3):877-92. Epub 2006 Mar 15.

19. John O. Clarke, MD, Gerard E. Mullin, MD A Review of Complementary and Alternative Approaches to Immunomodulation

20. Chistiakov DA. Immunogenetics of Hashimoto's thyroiditis. Journal of Autoimmune Diseases. 2005, 2:1

21. Xie LD, Gao Y, Li MR, Lu GZ, Huo XH. Distribution of immunoglobulin G subclasses of anti-thyroid peroxidase antibody in sera from patients with Hashimoto's thyroiditis with different thyroid functional status. Clinical and Experimental Immunology, 2008. 154: 172-176

22. Ganesh BG, Bhattachrya P, Gopisetty A, Prabhakar BS. Role of Cytokines in the Pathogenesis and Suppression of Thyroid Autoimmunity. Journal of Interferon and Cytokine Research. 2011; 31: 10: 721-731

23. Sanna Filén S. Lahesmaa R. GIMAP Proteins in T-Lymphocytes, Journal of Signal Transduction, vol. 2010, Article ID 268589, 10 pages, 2010. doi:10.1155/2010/268589

24. Hygiene Hypothesis. Accessed on 11/1/12 at: http://www.hygienehypothesis.com/

25. Zalctel K, Gaberscek S. Hashimoto's Thyroiditis: From Genes to Disease. Current Genomics, 2011, 12, 576-588

26. Nanba T, Watanabe M, Inoue N, Iwatani Y. Increases of the TH1/Th2 Ratio in Severe Hashimoto's Disease in the Proportion of Th17 Cells in Intractable Graves' Disease. Thyroid. 19, 5, 2009

27. CliffsNotes.com. Humoral and Cell-Mediated Immune Responses. 7 Nov 2012 http://www.cliffsnotes.com/study_guide/topicArticleId-277792,articleId-277723.html

28. http://chriskresser.com/basics-of-immune-balancing-for-hashimotos accessed 11/8/12

29. http://digitalnaturopath.com/cond/C104673.html accessed 11/8/12

30. http://www.easyhealthzone.com/autoimmune-diseases-s/30.htm accessed on 11/8/12

31. Peterson JD, Herzenberg LA, Vasquez K, Waltenbaugh C. Glutathione levels in antigen-presenting cells determine whether Th1 or Th2 response patterns predominate. Proc Natl Acad Sci USA 1998 Mar 17;95(6): pp.3071-6

32. www.lowdosenaltrexone.org accessed on 11/8/12

33. http://www.precisionnutrition.com/rr-green-tea-hazards accessed on 11/8/12

34. http://wellnessalternatives-stl.blogspot.com/2012/05/am-i-th1-or-th2-or-th17.html accessed on 11/8/12

35. http://www.youtube.com/watch?v=LSYED-7riNY&feature=related accessed on 11/8/12

36. http://articles.mercola.com/sites/articles/archive/2009/03/14/Clearing-Up-Confusion-on-Vitamin-D--Why-I-Dont-Recommend-the-Marshall-Protocol.aspx

37. Shoji J, Inada N, Sawa M.Antibody array-generated cytokine profiles of tears of patients with vernal keratoconjunctivitis or giant papillary conjunctivitis. Jpn J Ophthalmol. 2006 May-Jun;50(3):195-204.

38. Tamer G, Arik S, Tamer I, Coksert D. Relative Vitamim D Insufficiency in Hashimoto's thyroiditis. Thyroid 21(8), 2011

39. Sherry, er al. Sickness behavior induced by endotoxin can be mitigated by the dietary soluble fiber, pectin, through up-regulation of IL-4 and Th2 polarization. Brain Behav Immun. 2010 May; 24(4):631-640

40. Anatabine Investigator's Information. Rock Creek Pharmaceuticals. June 2012. www.anatabloc.com accessed 3/15/13

41. Gui J, Xiong F, Li J, Huang G. Effects of Acupuncture on Th1, Th2 Cytokines in Rats of Implantation Failure . Evidence-Based Complementary and Alternative MedicineVolume 2012 (2012)

42. XIE Changcai XU Nenggui DU Yixu Effect of Acupuncture on Th1/Th2 Cytokine Balance in Guinea Pigs with Alleraic Reaction TvpeIV. Journal of New Chinese Medicine, 5 (2008)

43. Jurenka, JS. Anti-inflammatory Properties of Curcumin, a Major Constituent of *Curcuma longa:* A Review of Preclinical and Clinical Research. *Altern Med Rev* 2009;14(2):141-153

44. Fujinami RS, von Herrath MG, Christen U, Whitton JL. Molecular mimicry, bystander activation or viral persistence: infection and autoimmune disease, Clinical microbiology reviews, Jan 2006 p 80-94

45. Vojdani A, Lambert J. The Role of Th17 in Neuroimmune Disorders. Target for CAM Therapy. Part II. Evidence Based Complementary and alternative medicine. Volume 1; 2011

46. Shi Y et. Al. Differentiation Imbalance of Th1/Th17 in Peripheral Blood mononuclear cells might contribute to pathogenesis of Hashimoto's thyroiditis. Scandinavian journal of immunology. 72, 250-255

47. Patarka, R. Cytokines and chronic fatigue syndrome. Ann N Y Acad Sci. 2001 Mar;933:185-200.

Chapter 11 References

1. Ulluwishewa, et.al. Regulation of Tight Junction Permeability by Intestinal Bacteria and Dietary Components. The Journal of Nutrition. March 23, 2011

2. Maes M, et;a. Increased serum IgA and IgM against LPS of enterbacteria in chronic fatigue syndrome (CFS): Indcation for the involvement of gram negative enterbacteria in the etiology og CFS and for the presence of an increased gut-intestinal permeability . Journal of Affective Disorders 99 (200&) 237-240

3. Maes M, Coucke F, Leunis JC. Normalization of increased translocation of endotoxin from gram-negative enterobacteria (Leaky gut) is accompanied by a remission of chronic fatigue syndrome Neuro Endocrinol Lett. 2007 28 (6):739-744

4. Maes M, Leunis JC. Normalization of leaky gut in chronic fatigue syndrome (CFS) is accompanied by a clinical improvement: effects of age, duration of illness and the translocation of LPS from gram-negative bacteria. Neuro Endocrinol Lett. 2008 Dec;29(6):902-10.

5. El-Tawil AM. Zinc supplementation tightens leaky gut in Crohn's disease. Inflamm Bowel Dis. 2012 Feb;18(2):E399. doi: 10.1002/ibd.21926. Epub 2011 Oct 12. PMID: 21994075

6. Lutgendorff F, Akkermans LM, Söderholm JD.The role of microbiota and probiotics in stress-induced gastro-intestinal damage. Curr Mol Med. 2008 Jun;8(4):282-98.

7. Maes, M, Mihaylova, I, De Ruyter, M. Lower Serum zinc in chronic fatigue syndrome (CFS): Relationship to immune dysfunctions and relevance for the oxidative stress status in CFS. Journal of Affective Disorders (2005)

8. Ulluwishewa D., et.al. Regulation of Tight Junction Permeability by Intestinal Bacteria and Dietary Components. The Journal of Nutrtion. 141: 769-776, 2011

9. Gibson GR, Beatty ER, Wang X, Cummings JH. Selective Stimulation of Bifidobacteria in the Human Colon by Oligofructose and Inulin. Gastroentorology. 1995; 108:975-982

10. Fasano A. Leaky Gut and autoimmune disease. Clin Rev Allergy Immunol. 2012 Feb;42(1):71-8.

11. Fasano A. Zonulin and Its Regulation of Intestinal Barrier Function: The

Biological Door to Inflammation, Autoimmunity, and Cancer. Physiol Rev. Vol 91. Jan 2011. 151-175

12. Patel RM, Myers LS, Kurundkar AR, Maheshwari A, Nusrat A, Lin PW. Probiotic bacteria induce maturation of intestinal claudin 3 expression and barrier function. Am J Pathol. 2012 Feb;180(2):626-35.

13. Rapin JR, Wiernsperger N. Possible links between intestinal permeablity and food processing: a potential therapeutic niche for glutamine. Clinics. 2010;65(6):635-43.

14. Vaarala O. Is the origin of type 1 diabetes in the gut? Immunol Cell Biol. 2012 Mar;90(3):271-6.

15. Vaarala O, Atkinson MA, Neu J. The "Perfect Storm" for Type 1 Diabetes: The Complex interplay between Intestinal Microbiota, Gut Permeability, and Mucosal Immunity. Diabetes 57:2555-2562, 2008

16. Campbell-McBride N. Gut and Psychology Syndrome. Halstan & Co. Ltd 2010

17. Gates, D. Body Ecology Diet. Hay House, Inc. 2011

18. Gibson GR, Macfarlane GT, Cummings JH. Sulphate reducing bacteria and hydrogen metabolism in the human large intestine. Gut 1993; 34: 437-439

19. http://bodyecology.com/articles/gut-permeability.php

20. Kirpich, Irina A (05/2012). "The type of dietary fat modulates intestinal tight junction integrity, gut permeability, and hepatic toll-like receptor expression in a mouse model of alcoholic liver disease". Alcoholism, clinical and experimental research (0145-6008), 36 (5), 835.

21. Wang, Hong-Bo (06/09/2012). "Butyrate Enhances Intestinal Epithelial Barrier Function via Up-Regulation of Tight Junction Protein Claudin-1 Transcription". Digestive diseases and sciences (0163-2116)

22. Benjamin J, Makharia G, Ahuja V, Joshi YK. Glutamine and Whey Protein Improve Intestinal Permeability and Morphology in Patients with Crohn's Disease: A Randomized Controlled TrialDig Dis Sci (2012) 57:1000–1012

23. Campbell-McBride N. Food Allergy. Journal of Orthomolecular Medicine, First Quarter, 2009, Vol 24, 1, pp.31-41 Available at http://gaps.me/preview/?page_id=344

24. Gottschall E. Breaking the vicious cycle. Intestinal health through diet. 1996. The Kirkton Press.

25. Vermeulen MAR, de Jong J, Vaessen MJ, van Leeuwen PAM, Houdijk APJ. Glutamate reduces experimental intestinal hyperpermeability and facilitates glutamine support of gut integrity. World J Gastroenterol. 2011 March 28: 17(12): 1569-1573

26. Rao, RK. Samak G. Role of Glutamine in Protection of Intestinal Epithelial Tight Junctions. Journal of Epithelial Biology and Pharmacology, 2012, 5 (Suppl 1-M7) 47-54

27. Pimentel M. Gut Microbes and Irritable Bowel Syndrome. IBS Centers for Educational Expertise, 2011

28. Pimentel M, Mayer A, Park S, Chow E, Hasan A, Kong Y. Methane production during lactulose test is associated with Gastrointestinal disease presentation. Digestive Diseases and Sciences, Vol 48, NO 1 (January 2003), pp 86-92

29. Mori, K. Does the gut microbiota Trigger Hashimoto's Disease? Discovery magazine, November 2012

30. Calcinaro F, Dionisi S, et. Al. Oral probiotic administration induces IL-10 production and prevents spontaneous autoimmune diabetes in no-obese diabetic mice. Diabetologia (2005) 48: 1565-1575

31. Kidd, PM. Multiple Sclerosis, an autoimmune inflammatory Disease: prospects for its integrative management. Alternative medicine Review. 6(6) 2001

32. Vyasm U, Ranganathan N. Probiotics, Prebiotics, and Symbiotic: Gut and Beyond. Gastroenterology Research and Practice. Volume 2012, Article ID 872716

33. Daher, R, Yazbeck T, Jaoude JB, Abboud B. Consequences of dysthyroidism on the digestive tract and viscera. World J Gastroenterol. 2009 June 21: 15(23)" 2834-2838h

34. Lakhan S, Kirchgessner A. Gut inflammation in chronic fatigue syndrome. Nutrition and Metabolism, 2010, 7:79

35. Rozalski A. May 2010 Potential virulence factors of Proteus bacilli. Journal of Microbiology and Molecular Biology, 61:65-89

36. Ebringer E, Khalafpour S, Wilson, C. Rheumatology International. Rheumatoid arthritis and proteus. a possible aetiological association. November 1989, Volume 9, Issue 3-5, pp 223-228

37. Struble K. July 2010. Journal of Pathophysiology Medscape. http://emedicine.medscape.com/article/226434-overview#a0104 Proteus vulgaris. Citizendium, 3 December 2010. Citizendium http://en.citizendium.org/wiki/Proteus_vulgaris

38. Koronakis V, Cross M, Senior B, Koronakis E, Hughes C. Journal of Bacteriology. April 1987, 169(4):1509-1515

39. Rashid, T. Ebringer A. Autoimmunity in Rheumatic Diseases Is Induced by Microbial Infections via Crossreactivity or Molecular Mimicry. Autoimmune Dis. 2012; 2012: 539282.

40. Effraimidis G, Tijssen JG, Strieder TG, Wiersinga WM. No causal relationship between Yersinia enterocolitica infection and autoimmune thyroid disease: evidence from a prospective study. Clin Exp Immunol. 2011 Jul;165(1):38-43.

41. Diagram of the Human Intestine. Drawn by Duncan Lock and released into the Public Domain. Available at http://commons.wikimedia.org/wiki/File:Intestine-diagram.svg Accessed March 29, 2013

42. Di Cagno R, et .al. Sourdough Bread Made from Wheat and Nontoxic Flours and Started with Selected Lactobacilli Is Tolerated in Celiac Sprue Patients. Appl Environ Microbiol. 2004 February; 70(2): 1088–1096.

43. Di Cagno R, et .al. Use of selected sourdough strains of Lactobacillus for removing gluten and enhancing the nutritional properties of gluten-free bread. J Food Prot. 2008 Jul;71(7):1491-5.

44. Moroni AV, Dal Bello F, Arendt EK. Sourdough in gluten-free bread-making: an ancient technology to solve a novel issue? Food Microbiol. 2009 Oct;26(7):676-84.

45. Gobbetti M, Giuseppe Rizzello C, Di Cagno R, De Angelis M. Sourdough lactobacilli and celiac disease. Food Microbiol. 2007 Apr;24(2):187-96. Epub 2006 Sep 12.

46. Di Cagno R, et .al. Gluten-free sourdough wheat baked goods appear safe for young celiac patients: a pilot study. J Pediatr Gastroenterol Nutr. 2010 Dec;51(6):777-83

Chapter 12 References

1. Bates, JM. Akerlund J, Mittge E, Guillemin K. Intestinal Alkaline Phosphatase Detoxifies Lipopolysaccharide and Prevents Inflammation in Response to the Gut Microbiota. Cell Host Microbe. 2007 December 13; 2(6): 371–382.

2. O'Grady JG et. al. Intestinal lactase, sucrase, and alkaline phosphatase in 373 patients with coeliac disease. J Clin Pathol 1984; 37:298-301

3. Jackson, SH. The effect of food ingestion on intestinal and serum alkaline phosphatase in rats. J. Biol. Chem. 1952; 553-559

4. Whitehead J. Intestinal alkaline phosphatase: The molecular link between rosacea and gastrointestinal disease. Medical Hypotheses 73 (2009) 1019-1022

5. Yang Y, Wandler AM, Postlethwait JH, Guillemin. Dynamic evolution of the LPS-detoxifying enzyme intestinal alkaline phosphatase in zebrafish and other vertebrates. Frontiers in Immunology. Oct 2012; 3(314) 1-15

6. Lalles JP. Intestinal alkaline phosphatase: multiple biological roles in maintenance of intestinal homeostasis and modulation by diet. Nutrition Reviews. Vol 68 (6): 323-332

7. Cheng YM, Ferreira P, Frohlich J, Schulzer M, Tan F. The effects of age, smoking, and alcohol on routine laboratory tests. Am J Clin Pathol. 1981 Mar;75(3):320-6.

8. Bayer PM, Hotschek H, Knoth E. Intestinal alkaline phosphatase and the ABP blood group system-a new aspect. Clin Chim Acta. 1980 NPv 20; 108(1): 81-7

9. Cui L, et. al. Prolonged zinc-deficient diet alters alkaline phosphatase and disaccharidase activities and induces morphological changes in the intestine of rats. The Journal of Trace Elements in Experimental Medicine 12/1998; 8(4):249 - 261.

10. Moreno J, Asteggiano CA, De Cattoni SD, Blanco A. Intestinal alkaline phosphatase: qualitative changes produced by deficient diet in rats. Metabolism. 1972 Jun;21(6):513-20.

11. Hansen GH, Rasmussen K, Niels-Christiansen LL, Danielsen EM. Dietary free fatty acids form alkaline phosphatase-enriched microdomains in the intestinal brush border membrane. Mol Membr Biol. 2011 Feb;28(2):136-44. Epub 2010 Dec 17.

12. Motzok I, McCuaig LW. Regulation of intestinal alkaline phosphatase by dietary phosphate. Can J Physiol Pharmacol. 1972 Dec;50(12):1152-6.

Chapter 13 References

1. Wilson, James. Adrenal Fatigue: The 21st Century Stress Syndrome. Smart Publications, 2011
2. Guilliams TG, Edwards L. Chronic Stress and The HPA Axis: Clinical Assessment and therapeutic Considerations. The Standard. Point Institute of Nutraceutical Research. 9 (2): 2012
3. Nieman, LK. Patient Information: Adrenal Insufficiency (Addison's Disease)(Beyond the Basics). In: uptodate, Lacroix, A, Martin KA (Ed), uptodate, Waltham, MA, 2011.
4. Nieman, LK. Causes of Primary Adrenal Insufficiency (Addison's Disease). In: uptodate, Lacroix, A, Martin KA (Ed), uptodate, Waltham, MA, 2012.
5. Nieman, LK. Pathogenesis of Adrenal Insufficiency In: uptodate, Lacroix, A, Martin KA (Ed), uptodate, Waltham, MA, 2012.
6. Adaptogens. In: Natural Standard: the authority on integrative medicine [database on the Internet]. Cambridge (MA): Natural Standard; 2012 [cited 5 December 2012]. Available from: http://www.naturalstandard.com. Subscription required to view.
7. Adrenal Extracts. In: Natural Standard: the authority on integrative medicine [database on the Internet]. Cambridge (MA): Natural Standard; 2012 [cited 5 December 2012]. Available from: http://www.naturalstandard.com. Subscription required to view.
8. DHEA. In: Natural Standard: the authority on integrative medicine [database on the Internet]. Cambridge (MA): Natural Standard; 2012 [cited 5 December 2012]. Available from: http://www.naturalstandard.com. Subscription required to view
9. Www.normshelley.com accessed 11/20/12
10. Wilder RL. Adrenal and gonadal steroid hormone deficiency in the pathogenesis of rheumatoid arthritis. J Rheumatol Suppl. 1996 Mar;44:10-2
11. Falorni A. Early Subclinical Addison's disease. Endocrine Abstracts (2009) 20 S9.3
12. Penev P, Spiegel K, Marcinkowski T, Van Cauter E. Impact of carbohydrate-rich meals on plasma epinephrine levels: dysregulation with aging. J Clin Endocrinol Metab. 2005 Nov;90(11):6198-206. Epub 2005 Aug 9.
13. Http://www.gisymbol.com.au/cmsadmin/uploads/Glycemic-Index-Foundation-Healthy-Choices-Brochure.pdf, accessed 11/20/12
14. Physician Road Map. Interpretive Guide and Suggested Protocols for the Adrenal Recovery Kit Adrenal Stress Profile. Ortho Molecular Products. Third Edition. Accessed on 11/21/12 at www.orthomolecularproducts.com Subscription required

15. Molina PE. Chapter 4. Thyroid Gland. In: Molina PE, ed. Endocrine Physiology. 3rd Ed. New York: Mcgraw-Hill; 2010. Http://www.accessmedicine.com/content.aspx?Aid=6169456. Accessed June 10th, 2012.
16. Fernando Lizcano, F, Rodríguez, JS. Thyroid hormone therapy modulates hypothalamo-pituitary- adrenal axis. Endocrine Journal 2011, 58 (2), 137-142
17. Hyman, M. The ultramind Solution: Companion Guide. Hyman Enterprises. 2009
18. Ross, DS. Central Hypothyroidism In: uptodate, Cooper DS, Mulder JE (Ed), uptodate, Waltham, MA, 2012.
19. Bhattacharyya A, Kaushal K, Tymms DJ, Davis JR. Steroid withdrawal syndrome after successful treatment of Cushing's syndrome: a reminder. Eur J Endocrinol. 2005 Aug;153(2):207-10.
20. Pavlaki AN, Magiakou MA, Chrousos GP. Chapter 14 – Glucocorticoid Therapy and Adrenal Suppression. Endotext. Accessed at http://www.endotext.org/adrenal/adrenal14/adrenalframe14.htm
21. Http://www.health-and-wisdom.com/store/p/1067-MAGNESIUM-OIL-64-OUNCE-PUMP-DISPENSER-SOLD-SEPARATELY-.aspx accessed 1/31/13
22. Adaptogens. In: Natural Standard: the authority on integrative medicine [database on the Internet]. Cambridge (MA): Natural Standard; 2012 [cited 5 December 2012]. Available from: http://www.naturalstandard.com. Subscription required to view
23. GIerach M, Gierach J, Skowronska A, Rutkowska E, Spychalska M, Pujanek M, Junik R. Hashimoto's thyroiditis and carbohydrate metabolism disorders in patients hospitalized in the Department of Endocrinology and Diabetology of Ludwik Rydigier Collegium Medicum in Bydgoszcz between 2001 and 20120. Polish Journal of Endocrinology, Vol 63, 1, 2012

Chapter 14 References

1. Loyola University Health System. "Increased Stroke Risk From Birth Control Pills, Review Finds." Science Daily, 27 Oct. 2009. Web. 26 Jan. 2013.
2. Cell Press. "Unnatural Selection: Birth Control Pills May Alter Choice Of Partners." ScienceDaily, 8 Oct. 2009. Web. 26 Jan. 2013.
3. Cohen S. Drug Muggers. Rodale. 2011
4. Nutrient Depletions in Natural Standard: the authority on integrative medicine [database on the Internet]. Cambridge (MA): Natural Standard; 2012 [cited 5 December 2012]. Available from: http://www.naturalstandard.com. Subscription required to view.
5. Shrader SP, Diaz VA. Chapter 88. Contraception. In: Talbert RL, DiPiro JT, Matzke GR, Posey LM, Wells BG, Yee GC, eds. Pharmacotherapy: A Pathophysiologic Approach. 8th ed. New York: McGraw-Hill; 2011.

http://0-
www.accesspharmacy.com.millennium.midwestern.edu/content.aspx?aID=
7993297. Accessed May 4, 2013.

6. Giron-Gonzalez JA, Moral FJ, Elvira J, Garcia-Gil D, Guerrero F, Gavilan, Escobar L. Consistent production of a higher TH1:TH2 cytokine ratio by stimulated T cells in men compared with women. European Journal of Endocrinology (2000) 143 31-36

7. Negro, R., Greco, G., Mangieri, T. et al. (2007) The influence of selenium supplementation on postpartum thyroid status in pregnant women with thyroid peroxidase autoantibodies. Journal of Clinical Endocrinology and Metabolism, 92, 1263–1268.

8. Giron-Gonzalez JA, Moral FJ, Elvira J, Garcia-Gil D, Guerrero F, Gavilan, Escobar L. Consistent production of a higher TH1:TH2 cytokine ratio by stimulated T cells in men compared with women. European Journal of Endocrinology (2000) 143 31-36

9. Drutel A, Archambeaud, F, Caron, P. Selenium and the thyroid gland. Clin Endocrinol. 2013;78(2):155-164.

10. Vestergaard P, Rejnmark L, Weeke J, Hoeck HC, Nielsen HK, Rungby J et al. Smoking as a risk factor for Graves' disease, toxic nodular goiter, and autoimmune hypothyroidism. Thyroid 2002 12 69 – 75

11. Ando T, Davies TF. Clinical Review 160: Postpartum autoimmune thyroid disease: the potential role of fetal microchimerism. J Clin Endocrinol Metab. 2003;88(7):2965.

12. Gottfried, S. The Hormone Cure. Scribner, 2013

13. Weschler T. Taking Charge of Your Fertility. Harper Collins; 2006

14. www.marshallprotocol.com and www.curemyTh1.org

15. Eschler DC, Hasham A, Tomer Y. Cutting edge: The etiology of autoimmune thyroid diseases. Clin Rev Allergy Immunol.2011 October; 41(2): 190-197

16. Desailloud R, Hober D. Viruses and thyroiditis: an update. Virol J 2009; 6: 5

17. The Antiadhesion Properties of Cranberries. www.cranberryinstitute.org Accessed 3/1/13

18. Patil BS, Patil S, Gururaj TR. Probable autoimmune causal relationship between periodontitis and Hashimotos thyroiditis: A systemic Review. Nigerian Journal of Clinical Practice, Jul-Sep 2011. Vol 14 (3) p253

19. Fluoride Linked to Gum Disease.
http://www.medicalnewstoday.com/releases/71584.php accessed 4/22/13

20. Vananda, KL, Sesha Reddy M. Indian J Dent Res 2007. 18(2): 67-71

Chapter 15 References

1. Guo H, Jiang T, Wang J, Chang Y, Guo H, Zhang W. The value of eliminating foods according to food-specific immunoglobulin G antibodies in irritable bowel syndrome with diarrhoea. J Int Med Res 2012;40(1):204-10.

2. Danivic J.N. Ramirez, MD, Vergara-Villaluz JC, Lagdameo-Leuenberger MP, Jasul GV, Añel-Quimpo, JA. Prevalence of Thyroid Dysfunction Among

Individuals Taking Glutathione Supplementation: A Cross-Sectional Study Preliminary Report. Phillipne Journal of Internal medicine. Volume 48 Number 3 Oct.-Dec., 2010

3. Biesiekierski JR, Newnham ED, Irving PM, Barrett JS, Haines M, Doecke JD et al. Gluten causes gastrointestinal symptoms in subjects without celiac disease: a double-blind randomized placebo-controlled trial. AM J Gastroenterol (2010) 106: 508-514

4. Suen RM, Gordon S. A Critical Review of IgG Immunoglobulins and Food Allergy-Implications in Systemic Health. Us BioTek Laboratories, 2003

5. Lambert SE, Kinder JM, Then JE, Parliament KN, Bruns HA. Erythromycin treatment hinders the induction of oral tolerance to fed ovalbumin. Frontiers in Immunology. July 2012

6. Ensminger. Allergies. Food and Nutrition Encyclopedia; CRC Press. 1994

7. Lipski, L. Digestive Wellness. McGraw-Hill Publishing, 2011

Chapter 16 References

1. Connett P, Beck J, Micklem HS. The case against fluoride: How hazardous waste ended up in our drinking water and the bad science and powerful politics that keep it there. Chelsea Green, VT, 2010

2. De Coster S, van Larebeke N. Endocrine-disrupting chemicals: associated disorders and mechanisms of action. J Environ Public Health. 2012;2012:713696. Epub 2012 Sep 6.

3. http://www.ewg.org/research/down-drain/what-you-can-do

4. Bahn AK, Mills JL, Snyder PJ, Gann PH, Houten L, Bialik O, Jollman L, Utiger RD. Hypothyroidism in workers exposed to polybrominated biphenyls. N Engl J Med. 1980 Jan 3; 302(1):31-3

5. http://www.nontoxicbeds.com/

6. Eschler DC, Hasham A, Tomer Y. Cutting edge: The etiology of autoimmune thyroid diseases. Clin Rev Allergy Immunol.2011 October; 41(2): 190-197)

7. Cross DW, Carton RJ (2003). "Fluoridation: a violation of medical ethics and human rights". International Journal of Occupational and Environmental Health 9 (1): 24–9.

8. http://chemistry.about.com/od/chemistryhowtoguide/a/removefluoride.htm

9. Bachinskii PP et al. 1985. Action of the body fluorine of healthy persons and thyroidopathy patients on the function of hypophyseal-thyroid the system. *Probl Endokrinol (Mosk)* 31(6):25-9. [See study]

10. Burgi H, et al. (1984). Fluorine and the Thyroid Gland: A Review of the Literature. *Klin Wochenschr.* 1984 Jun 15;62(12):564-9.

11. Caldwell KL, et al. (2008). Iodine status of the U.S. population, National Health and Nutrition Examination Survey 2003-2004. *Thyroid* 18(11):1207-14.

12. Choi AL, et al. (2012). Developmental Fluoride Neurotoxicity: A Systematic Review and Meta-Analysis. *Environmental Health Perspectives* 2012 Jul 20. [Epub ahead of print]

13. Hosur MB, et al. (2012). Study of thyroid hormones free triiodothyronine (FT3), free thyroxine (FT4) and thyroid stimulating hormone (TSH) in subjects with dental fluorosis. European Journal of Dentistry 6:184-90.
14. Klein RZ, et al. (2010). Relation of severity of maternal hypothyroidism to cognitive development of offspring. Journal of Medical Screening 8(1):18-20.
15. Haddow JE, et al. (1999). Maternal thyroid deficiency during pregnancy and subsequent neuropsychological development of the child. New England Journal of Medicine 341(8):549-55.
16. Lin F, et al (1991). The relationship of a low-iodine and high-fluoride environment to subclinical cretinism in Xinjiang. Endemic Disease Bulletin 6(2):62-67 (republished in Iodine Deficiency Disorder Newsletter Vol. 7(3):24-25). [See study]
17. Lin F, et al. (1986). A preliminary approach to the relationship of both endemic goiter and fluorosis in the valley of Manasi River, Xin-Jiang to environmental geochemistry. Chinese Journal of Endemiology 5(1):53-55.
18. Maumené E. (1854). Experiencé pour déterminer l'action des fluores sur l'economie animale. Compt Rend Acad Sci *(Paris)* 39:538-539.
19. Mikhailets ND, et al. (1996). Functional state of thyroid under extended exposure to fluorides Probl Endokrinol (Mosk) 42:6-9. [See study]
20. National Research Council. (2006). Fluoride in drinking water: a scientific review of EPA's standards. National Academies Press, Washington D.C. [See study]
21. Pontigo-Loyola A, et al. (2008). Dental fluorosis in 12- and 15-year-olds at high altitudes in above-optimal fluoridated communities in Mexico. Journal of Public Health Dentistry 68(3):163-66.
22. Susheela AK, et al. (2005). Excess fluoride ingestion and thyroid hormone derangements in children living in New Delhi, India. *Fluoride* 38:98-108. [See study]
23. http://www.fluoridealert.org/issues/health/thyroid/
24. Beierwaltes, WH, Nishiyama RH. Dog thyroiditis: occurrence and similarity to Hashimoto's Struma. Endocrinology 1968 83: 501-508;
25. Basha PM, Rai P, Begum S. Fluoride toxicity and status of serum thyroid hormones, brain histopathology, and learning memory in rats: a multigenerational assessment. Biol Trace Elem Res. 2011 Dec;144(1-3):1083
26. Zeng Q, Cui YS, Zhang L, Fu G, Hou CC, Zhao L, Wang AG, Liu HL. Studies of fluoride on the thyroid cell apoptosis and mechanism. 2012 Mar;46(3):233-6.
27. http://thyroid.about.com/od/drsrichkarileeshames/a/fluoride2006.htm
28. Nabrzyski M, Gajewska R - "Aluminium and fluoride in hospital daily diets and in teas" Z Lebensm Unters Forsch 201(4):307-10 (1995)
29. http://www.ewg.org/foodnews/summary/
30. http://chemistry.about.com/od/chemistryhowtoguide/a/removefluoride.htm
31. http://www.fluoridealert.org/faq/
32. http://www.fluoridealert.org/content/water_filters/
33. http://www.slweb.org/ftrcfluorinatedpharm.html
34. http://www.ewg.org/guides/cleaners

35. Brent, GA. Environmental Exposures and Autoimmune Thyroid Disease. Thyroid. 2010 July; 20(7): 755–761.
36. Lee AN, Werth VP. Activation of autoimmunity following use of immunostimulatory herbal supplements. Arch Dermatol. 2004 Jun;140(6):723
37. Detoxification. In: Natural Standard: the authority on integrative medicine [database on the Internet]. Cambridge (MA): Natural Standard; 2012 [cited 5 December 2012]. Available from: http://www.naturalstandard.com. Subscription required to view.

Chapter 17 References

1. https://www.aarda.org/q_and_a.php accessed on 4/1/13

Chapter 18 References

1. Daniel, Kaayla. The Healing Power of Broth. Accessed at http://www.thenourishinggourmet.com/2011/09/the-healing-power-of-broth.html
2. Bosscher D, Breynaert A, Pieters L, Hermans N. Food-based strategies to modulate the composition of the intestinal microbiota and their associated health effects. Journal of Physiology and Pharmacology 2009; 60, Suppl 6, 5-11
3. Barrett JS, Gibson PR. Fermentable oligosaccharides, disaccharides, monosaccharides and polyols (FODMAPs) and nonallergic food intolerance: FODMAPs or food chemicals. The Adv Gastroenterol (2012) 5(4) 261-268
4. http://thyroidbook.com/blog/autoimmune-gut-repair-diet/
5. Carroccio A, Mansueto P, Iacono G, Soresi M, D'Alcamo A, Cavataio F, Brusca I, Florena AM, Ambrosiano G, Seidita A, Pirrone G, Rini GB. Non-celiac wheat sensitivity diagnosed by double-blind placebo-controlled challenge: exploring a new clinical entity. Am J Gastroenterol. 2012 Dec;107(12):1898-906;
6. Dugdale DC. Low Residue Fiber Diet. Medline. http://www.nlm.nih.gov/medlineplus/ency/patientinstructions/000200.htm acessed on 2/13/2013
7. Dulloo, A G (10/2011). "The search for compounds that stimulate thermogenesis in obesity management: from pharmaceuticals to functional food ingredients". *Obesity reviews (1467-7881)*, 12 (10), 866.
8. http://www.todaysdietitian.com/newarchives/072710p30.shtml
9. http://www.ibsgroup.org/brochures/fodmap-intolerances.pdf
10. Gottschall E. Breaking the vicious cycle. Intestinal health through diet. 1996. The Kirkton Press.
11. Campbell-McBride, N. Gut and Psychology Syndrome. Medinform Publishing, 2012.
12. Gates D, Schatz L. Body Ecology Diet. Hay House, 2011.
13. Mercola, J. This Food Contains 100 TIMES More Probiotics than a Supplement Accessed on 4/1/13 at: http://articles.mercola.com/sites/articles/archive/2012/05/12/dr-campbell-

mcbride-on-gaps.aspx
14. http://chefambershea.com/2012/04/03/coming-clean-my-battle-with-hashimotos-disease/ accessed 4/1/13

Chapter 19 References

1. McClain CJ,et. Al. Zinc status before and after zinc supplementation of eating disorder patients J Am Coll Nutr. 1992 Dec;11(6):694-700.
2. Naranjo CA, Busto U, Sellers EM et al. (1981). "A method for estimating the probability of adverse drug reactions". Clin. Pharmacol. Ther. **30** (2): 239–45

Chapter 20 References

1. Dell'edera, Domenico (08/2013). "Effect of multivitamins on plasma homocysteine in patients with the 5,10 methylenetetrahydrofolate reductase C677T homozygous state". Molecular medicine reports (1791-2997), 8 (2), 609.
2. McNulty, Helene (10/2012). "Nutrition throughout life: folate". International journal for vitamin and nutrition research (0300-9831), 82 (5), 348.
3. www.mthfr.net accessed 6/1/2013
4. Zappacosta, Bruno, et. al. "Homocysteine lowering by folate-rich diet or pharmacological supplementations in subjects with moderate hyperhomocysteincmia". Nutrients (2072-6643), 5 (5), 1531.
5. Prinz-Langenohl, R.; Brämswig, S.; Tobolski, O.; Smulders, Y.M.; Smith, D.E.C.; Finglas, P.M.; Pietrzik, K. [6S]-5-methyltetrahydrofolate increases plasma folate more effectively than folic acid in women with the homozygous or wildtype 677C→T polymorphism of methylenetetrahydrofolate reductase. Br. J. Pharmacol. **2009,** 158, 2014–2021
6. Prinz-Langenohl, R et.al. [6S]-5-methyltetrahydrofolate increases plasma folate more effectively than folic acid in women with the homozygous or wild-type 677C-->T polymorphism of methylenetetrahydrofolate reductase. British journal of pharmacology (0007-1188), 158 (8), 2014.
7. http://ods.od.nih.gov/factsheets/Folate-HealthProfessional/ accessed 6/3/13
8. http://ods.od.nih.gov/factsheets/VitaminB6-HealthProfessional/ accessed 6/3/13
9. https://www.mymedlab.com/autism/gi-effects-complete-mmx2100 accessed 6/3/13
10. http://www.metametrix.com/test-menu/profiles/gastrointestinal-function/dna-stool-analysis-gi-effects?t=clinicianInfo accessed 6/3/13
11. www.mylabsforlife.com accessed 6/3/13
12. www.zrtlabs.com accessed 6/3/13
13. Walsh, Nancy Folic acid caner debate continues, accessed 6/3/13 at http://www.medpagetoday.com/HematologyOncology/ColonCancer/37008
14. http://foodallergy.com/tests.html accessed 6/3/13

Index

ABOUT THE AUTHOR

Dr. Izabella Wentz, Pharm.D., FASCP is a pharmacist who has had a passion for health care from a very early age, inspired by her mother, Dr. Marta Nowosadzka, MD.

After being diagnosed with Hashimoto's Thyroiditis in 2009, Dr. Wentz was surprised at the lack of knowledge about lifestyle interventions for Hashimoto's and autoimmune conditions. She decided to take on lifestyle interventions as a personal mission in an effort to help herself and others with the same condition.

She has summarized three years of research and two years of testing in her book: "Hashimoto's Thyroiditis: Lifestyle Interventions for Finding and Treating the Root Cause." She currently lives in Chicago, IL, with her husband Michael and their dog Boomer, where she works as a medication safety pharmacist.

Dr. Wentz also has a small private practice and is available for consultations in person and via phone.

www.thyroidrootcause.org
www.thyroidlifestyle.com

Made in the USA
San Bernardino, CA
01 March 2016